Praise
*Your Natural M*

"*Your Natural Medicine Cabinet* is spot on with the most effective natural remedies that will help to heal and soothe everyday ailments. Having worked with one of Burke's mentors many years ago, I can now understand why she is so accomplished at arriving at the correct remedy for so many issues. This is one gem of a book that I wouldn't hesitate to recommend to all drug-free solution seekers."
— ANN LOUISE GITTLEMAN, PhD, CNS, *New York Times* bestselling author of 30 books on health and healing

"A super user-friendly introduction to the best and safest natural remedies that should be in everyone's medicine cabinet ... and how to use them to treat the most frequently experienced ailments. Full of good, practical information along with compelling personal stories. This book should be in every home!"
— DANA ULLMAN, MPH, author of 10 books on natural and homeopathic medicine

"This treasure trove of practical remedies is so well-written and understandable that it will appeal to a wide audience. Lennihan's years of experience and her knowledge of the literature that evaluates holistic approaches makes this a perfect addition to one's home library."
— JUDY NORSIGIAN, bestselling author of *Our Bodies, Ourselves*

"This valuable book makes it easy and enjoyable to find what you need to heal yourself naturally."
— PEGGY HUDDLESTON, author of *Prepare for Surgery, Heal Faster: A Guide of Mind-Body Techniques*

"*Your Natural Medicine Cabinet* has quickly become our top recommendation, the 'go-to book' for folks who want to know more about healing themselves. Packed with information running the gamut from a quick fix for small problems to longer-term use of supplements for all kinds of conditions, this book is a very enjoyable read. As a certified nutritionist and the owner of a health food store for nearly 40 years, I am truly impressed with Burke Lennihan's book and recommend it to our customers for the quick, easy-to-access, and vital information she puts out for her readers."
— ELIZABETH STAGL, CN, MS NutSci, co-owner of Cambridge Naturals, Cambridge, Mass.

"A tried-and-true natural medicine expert has pulled together a wealth of information anyone can easily understand and implement. This book is a treasure of resources you will be glad you have when illness strikes or you just want to be the healthiest you can be."

— JUNE RIEDLINGER SHIBLEY, RPh, PharmD, ND, former director of the Center for Integrative Therapies in Pharmaceutical Care, Massachusetts College of Pharmacy and Health Sciences

# *Your*
# NATURAL
# MEDICINE
# CABINET

———◆———

A PRACTICAL GUIDE TO DRUG-FREE
REMEDIES FOR COMMON AILMENTS

## Burke Lennihan

**GREEN HEALING PRESS**
Cambridge, Mass.

For information, address:
GreenHealing Press
777 Concord Ave., Suite 301
Cambridge, MA 02138
www.YourNaturalMedicineCabinet.com
E-mail: Burke@YourNaturalMedicineCabinet.com

For foreign and translation rights, contact Nigel J. Yorwerth
E-mail: Nigel@PublishingCoaches.com

Distributed by SCB Distributors
15608 South New Century Dr., Gardena, CA 90248
www.SCBDistributors.com
info@SCBDistributors.com

Library of Congress Control Number: 2012940857

ISBN: 978-0-9834430-2-5

10 9 8 7 6 5 4 3 2 1

Cover design: Nita Ybarra
Interior design: Alan Barnett

On the cover: Ginkgo biloba, one of the most ancient trees on earth,
has long been used in Traditional Chinese Medicine and more recently
in Western herbalism and homeopathy. Its usefulness in conventional
medicine has been documented by dozens of scientific trials.

This book is intended to serve only as a resource and informational
guide. It is not intended nor should it be taken as medical advice.
Individual readers are not engaged in individual therapy with either the
author or the publisher. The ideas, procedures, and suggestions in this
book are not intended as a substitute for consulting a professional.
All matters regarding health require medical supervision. Please consult
the section on "What's Safe to Treat at Home" for additional guidelines.
Neither the author nor the publisher shall be liable or responsible for
any loss, injury, or damage allegedly arising from any information or
suggestion in this book. The opinions expressed in this book represent
the personal views of the author.

*To Sri Chinmoy, my spiritual teacher,*
*who taught by his own radiant example*
*that a healthy body creates a dynamic vessel*
*for a peaceful, meditative life*

*and to my parents—*
*my father the doctor and my mother the teacher,*
*nature lovers both,*
*who gave me a wildflower garden when I was little*
*and with it a love for the healing powers of plants.*

# CONTENTS

**Part Three: Stocking Your Natural Medicine Cabinet**

**Part Four: How to Use Homeopathic Medicines**

**Part Five: Your Support System**

# DISCOVERING
# NATURAL HEALING

"Can it really work that fast?"

My running buddy's eyes were wide with astonishment. I had just dropped a natural remedy into her mouth and the pain from her cramps dissolved along with the pellets. We had just passed my health food store when she told me she had to turn around because her cramps were so bad. I suggested experimenting with something from the store. It was worth a try—it would be harmless at worst, and at best it might save our Saturday morning run. In fact the remedy worked almost instantaneously, as they sometimes do, and I was as astonished as she was.

It was one of the "ah ha moments" that led me to write this book. I spent 15 years working in the supplement department of my health food store, talking to my customers about what worked for them and focusing on:

∾ What works the best and fastest for common home-care conditions.

∾ What's safe and cost-effective for the family medicine cabinet.

∾ What's the simplest approach, one that anyone can master.

The result is this book. I hope it will empower you to create your own natural medicine cabinet. By treating everyday complaints at home, you'll stay healthier overall, you'll save time and money by preventing unnecessary trips to your primary care doctor or emergency room, and you'll lose less time from work for yourself or a sick child.

## How This Book Came About

This is probably the first crowd-sourced book in natural healing, with the "crowd" being my thousands of customers and clients going back to 1977 when I opened my health food store. Boston's historic Beacon Hill section in the late '70s housed blueblooded Brahmins in 18th century mansions and hippies in seedy apartments on the back side of the Hill. Tourists came from all over the world, drawn by the charm of the Revolutionary War-era brick buildings and the nearby Public Gardens.

In the '80s, gentrification brought yuppies to replace the hippies. With several distinguished colleges nearby, there were always students and professors. Mass. General Hospital was just a few blocks away, and surprisingly enough, some of its doctors and nurses ventured into my store along with staff members and patients' families. Dean Ornish was a lunchtime regular during his residency at Mass. General in the early '80s. My brick storefront, with its mullion-paned bay window painted a sunny yellow, was a magnet for granola-crunching humanity.

In the late '80s I moved the store across the river to West Cambridge, among the spacious Victorians near Fresh Pond. My new customers included Harvard faculty, writers, architects, lawyers, and doctors. The store was small (a "mom and pop" store without the "pop"— just me), so I worked at the checkout counter next to the supplement department by day and baked the cookies after the store closed at night. It was easy to get to know my customers, and I specialized in ordering supplements that they couldn't find anywhere else. I would always ask them what it was for, why it was better than what I already had on hand, and how they could tell that it worked.

In a small store (the Beacon Hill store was only 267 square feet and it included a vegetarian cafe!), I had to keep discarding run-of-the-mill supplements to make way for these new special finds. The result was the physical version of what you're holding in printed form: a few top recommendations for dozens of conditions. And because I catered to busy professionals with high-power jobs, the supplements also had to work quickly.

You'll notice, though, that I haven't limited myself to just one recommendation per condition. I found in my years in the store that just as some customers liked our maple walnut cookies soft on the inside and others wanted them crispy, so too did people have preferences in supplements. Some liked herbs, others liked vitamins, and among those who preferred herbs, some wanted convenient blends in capsules while others wanted to make their own teas and salves. Some wanted the best no matter what the cost, while others were willing to spend time preparing their own blends to save money.

So this book is drawn from the needs, preferences, and feedback of my customers in more than 15 years of running the store, and my clients in the more recent 15 years of holistic practice.

## My Journey in Natural Healing

I always wanted to be a doctor like my father. I came from a medical family: my father was a vascular surgeon who tested the very first Doppler ultrasound machine in his research lab, my mother was a biochemist who researched stains for Dr. Papanicolau while he developed the Pap smear, and my great-aunt was the chief nurse in the famous series of surgeries mapping the human brain. Dad was a sought-after speaker for stop-smoking groups, and he practiced his lectures on us at the dinner table complete with slides of gangrenous toes. (I never inhaled.)

But as an undergraduate I read Adelle Davis' *Let's Eat Right to Keep Fit* and discovered that chronic disease could be prevented, even treated, with healthy food and supplements instead of drugs and surgery. I became passionate about natural healing long before there were any schools offering professional training.

So it was that I graduated from Harvard and, in a truly unusual career move, opened a health food store. In search of answers for my customers' questions—what do you have for sore throats? for urinary tract infections? for insomnia?—I read voraciously, attended seminars led by pioneering natural healers, and learned from my customers' experience. In the shadow of Harvard and MIT, I had probably the most highly educated clientele of any health food store in the country.

One section of my store baffled me, however. I carried homeo-pathic remedies because people asked for them, but I found them mys-tifying. Very few customers seemed to know about them, but those who did reported amazing results. Homeopathy seemed to be a secret club known only to its initiates. When I had my "ah-ha" moment, I saw first-hand what these homeopathy aficionados had been telling me about apparently miraculous results which actually followed the laws of an obscure science.

On turning 40, I decided to pursue professional training in homeo-pathy. I wanted to master this arcane science not only to help indi-vidual clients with its safe and effective remedies, but more importantly to teach it widely in a simple and empowering way. I was fortunate to learn from Dr. Luc De Schepper, an internationally distinguished homeopath, and even more fortunate to help him found a school and write a handbook for home prescribers and a textbook for professionals. In the process I received the benefit of his accumulated experience from treating, in his long career and by his own estimation, more than 100,000 patients.

I now have the benefit of practicing homeopathy at the Lydian Center for Innovative Medicine in Cambridge, Mass. My colleagues include chiropractors, neuro-acupressure practitioners, a naturopath, and a craniosacral practitioner/Brain Gym expert. Some of my col-leagues are doing cutting-edge work in their fields, and we learn from each other as we share clients with challenging health problems. Our clients include Nobel laureates, professors at Harvard Medical School, physicians at Harvard teaching hospitals, and soloists at Boston Sym-phony Hall (or the families of these professionals). Many have done their own extensive internet search on their condition. I am humbled by how much my clients know about natural approaches to their health problems and I continue to learn from them.

In my own homeopathy practice since 1996, I have never forgotten my roots in my health food store. I recommend not only homeopathic medicines but also vitamins, herbs, changes in diet, perhaps another healing modality for my clients to pursue, and books to empower them by expanding their knowledge.

## How to Use This Book

My goal is to empower people to care for themselves and their families with the best natural products for many common conditions. "Best" sometimes means quickest, and quickest often means a homeopathic remedy. (For the skeptics, I review the latest research on how it works in Part Four—but this book is about what works, and in my experience homeopathy often works best. Try it, following the guidelines in Part Four, and decide for yourself.) Homeopathy can't work in isolation, though. It gives instructions, like providing the architect's drawings for a house, but you still need the "building materials" from supplements and superfoods.

The core of the book draws from my knowledge of supplements, homeopathic remedies, herbs, flower essences, cell salts, and superfoods. For each one I recommend a Quick Fix for immediate relief plus supportive supplements and lifestyle recommendations to provide ongoing relief or to prevent recurrence. Sometimes I recommend specific brands, most notably for herbs because some brands have powerful medicinal effects while others are basically worthless (depending on how carefully the herbs are handled). For homeopathic remedies, on the other hand, there is much less variation among brands because the FDA oversees homeopathic manufacturers, holding them to exacting standards. As for supplements, I recommend some by brand name, but there are other excellent brands and your local health food store staff can guide you.

Please don't skip over the first section, though. Your natural medicine cabinet will work best if you have a strong body to begin with. The suggestions in Part One are meant to be succinct and not overwhelming, yet to provide you with plenty of resources if you would like to know more about a particular topic.

In a world of information overload, I've tried to keep this book short, simple and empowering. I've also narrowed down the list of books and internet resources. (Web-based information about natural healing is often truly awful or overly commercialized.) While the recommended books and websites may seem like a lot, I certainly don't expect anyone to explore all or even most of them. Just start with one or two that interest you most.

In teaching this material to hundreds of students in my homeopathy school, I've found that it helps to present the information more than once, and from fresh angles. So while Part Two is arranged by condition, in Part Three I cut the deck differently: it's arranged by natural healing substances, beginning with a dozen or so that I would recommend having on hand right from the start.

Part Four, the section on how to use homeopathic medicines, really makes this book unique. In my health food store, the customers who knew how to use homeopathy got dramatic results, but others who were unfamiliar with it were often disappointed. Learning to use homeopathic remedies effectively is a bit like learning to ride a bike: there's some wobbling at first but then it becomes second nature. From years of teaching homeopathy, fielding questions from beginners, and observing where they tend to go off course, I've come up with a simple guide to using these natural medicines effectively. I encourage you to read it before you use any of the homeopathic medicines recommended in Part Two. A small effort to master the method will be well rewarded.

Part Five addresses one of the pitfalls I've noticed over the years among my clients and students. They often begin with tremendous enthusiasm for natural healing but then face skepticism from friends, family members, and health care practitioners. When they tell me about the criticism they've encountered, I usually find it's based on misunderstandings and misinformation about natural healing in general and homeopathy in particular.

Part of the solution is to provide good information you can use to respond to these critiques, as you'll see in Part Five. Another solution is to tell you about sources of support. You explorers in natural healing are not alone. Many of my clients, especially are mothers of small children, will say, "I feel like I'm the *only one* who is trying to keep my kids off sugar, limit TV and computer time, and avoid antibiotics if possible." Now with groups like HolisticMoms.org and Meetup groups, they're finding like-minded people to share enthusiasm, encouragement, and great information.

It's also important to find health care providers who are respectful of your choices. At the same time, we need to be respectful of mainstream health care providers and all their hard-won knowledge. Part Five recommends finding a doctor you can partner with, one who listens to you respectfully. It also gives guidance on finding a holistic health care professional trained to treat *chronic* illness, which is far beyond the scope of this book. Please note the guidelines at the beginning of Part Two on what's safe to treat at home versus when you really do need to call your doctor or go to the ER.

*Your Natural Medicine Cabinet* is meant as a handbook—a book to be taken in hand, to be manageable, to empower you with just the right amount of information rather than overwhelming you with too much. It's meant to make you feel that *yes*, you can do it: you *can* create a natural medicine cabinet and use it wisely for yourself and your family.

It's not meant to be encyclopedic. I've found that too much information is overwhelming for people new to natural healing, and too often people just give up without even trying. If you like this book and want to know more about supplements, please get Balch's *Prescription for Natural Cures* and *The Encyclopedia of Natural Medicine* by Pizzorno and Murray. I started recommending these books twenty years ago in my health food store and I continue to recommend them to my clients today. They are the definitive works in the field and will give you plenty of information.

This book is also not meant to cover chronic diseases like eczema, hypothyroidism and diabetes. You'll need professional help to turn those conditions around, although there's lots you can do with healthy food and supplements (see the resources in Part One) while searching for a holistic practitioner (as described in Part Five). Just a few chronic conditions (like arthritis, gout, and osteoporosis) are included because home care with food and supplements is so essential for treating them.

I have not attempted to cover Traditional Chinese Medicine or Ayurvedic healing in this book because I am not an expert in them, although I have great respect for the ancient healing systems of China and India. Different healing systems work for different people, and I encourage you to pursue these Eastern therapies if you feel drawn to them.

I'm sure you'll have questions. Please email me questions of *general* interest to **Burke@YourNaturalMedicineCabinet.com**, and I'll answer them in my blog on my website, **www.YourNaturalMedicineCabinet .com**. Email me your success stories if you'd like to share them (anonymously if you prefer). Keep checking the blog for updates, new natural products, and the latest research on natural healing. Welcome to the journey of natural healing!

**Notes:** I have no financial interest in any of the books or products I recommend (except the books and video seminars produced by GreenHealing Press). A portion of the proceeds from the sale of GreenHealing products goes to the GreenHealing Initiative, which shares the knowledge of natural healing with low-income families.

Sometimes I specify particular product brands because I've found in my many years in health care that these brands work very well. If I don't specify a brand, please choose any good health food store brand. (It's not worth trying to save money on cut-rate supplements, because their cheaper ingredients don't work as well in your body). When I have put the brand name of a product in **bold,** it means it is a unique formula and is not interchangeable with other similar products. There are many good brands, though, and if your local health food store doesn't have the one I mention here, please simply follow their recommendations.

I have changed details in the stories in this book to protect the privacy of those involved. The stories are all authentic and the direct quotes are accurate to the best of my memory. For readability throughout the text, I have capitalized the first letters of words in website addresses.

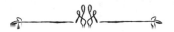

## Part One

# CREATING A STRONG FOUNDATION

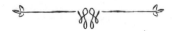

The suggestions in this section will create a strong foundation which will enable the recommendations in Part Two to work well. In particular, the "Preventing Recurrence" and "Lifestyle Support" suggestions in Part Two assume you're already doing what's recommended here.

True health means wellness on all levels — mental, emotional, and spiritual as well as physical health. You'll find suggestions in these areas as well.

# BOTTOM-LINE BASICS
# FOR HEALTHY EATING

These are the top health tips I've shared with my clients over the years. While there are many approaches to healthy eating, these are principles that most experts would agree on.

**Eat richly colored fruits and vegetables.** Your deep red and purple and orange fruits, your dark green and yellow vegetables, have the most nutrients because the pigments are the nutrients.

If you have any doubts about the healing power of these foods, check out the YouTube video of Dr. Terry Wahls' TED talk on how she cured herself of MS. As a physician, she had access to the best of conventional medical care, but was wheelchair-bound and getting worse. Then she researched the nutrients her body needed and how to get them from food. (The short version: lots and lots of vegetables!)

The "white food" exception: You've probably heard that it's best to avoid white foods: white bread, white sugar, white pasta. I agree. They're a waste of stomach space. Recent research has documented a few exceptions, though. The white fruits—pears and apples—seem to help prevent strokes; and white button mushrooms apparently have healing properties just like their darker cousins, the shiitake and maitake mushrooms.

**Get a Vita-Mix and make green smoothies.** A Vita-Mix (a super-duper, high-power blender) is perfect for busy lifestyles and fussy kids.

You can make fresh smoothies in a matter of minutes with raw fruits and vegetables. There's something about a Vita-Mix that turns green vegetables into a frothy, foamy, luscious treat. Green smoothies are delicious, and you can chug them while you're running out the door or driving to work. Amazingly, kids tend to like them. Get Victoria Boutenko's *Green Smoothie Revolution* and check out her how-to videos on YouTube.

I've given my clients many recommendations over the years, and I've received more positive feedback about this one than everything else put together. As with all products I recommend, I have no financial interest in Vita-Mix blenders or Victoria Boutenko's books.

**Eat healthy fats.** Surprisingly, coconut is now acknowledged as one of the healthiest. Try the So Delicious brand of coconut milk, yogurt and ice cream. Avocados have good quality fats and add a wonderful rich "mouth feel" to smoothies. Remember to buy oils in small quantities and keep them refrigerated (except you'll keep a small bottle of olive oil at room temperature because it hardens in the fridge). Oils get rancid easily when exposed to the air, and rancid oils are destructive to the fats in your body. That also means keeping nuts in the freezer.

**Treasure the tiny precious seeds.** The oils of certain tiny seeds — flax, evening primrose, hemp, borage, chia — are concentrated sources of wonderful oils. Recent research indicates that these "parent essential oils" may be even better for our body than fish oil. These seeds and their oils need to be handled carefully. The oils should be in an opaque black bottle and refrigerated after opening. The seeds should be bought whole and kept in the freezer. Buying the seeds already ground is not a good idea because as soon as those precious essential oils are exposed to air, they start to go rancid. Instead, grind the seeds in a coffee bean grinder or your new Vita-Mix just prior to using.

**Ditch the microwave.** It alters the molecules of your food so your body no longer recognizes them as nutrients. Plus it emits harmful radiation. (How did this device ever get a safety clearance from the government?) Not only does the food end up less nutritious, it can also develop cancer-causing compounds. Don't believe me? Read *Zapped* by Ann Louise Gittleman, a highly recommended resource.

Case in point: a colleague with a busy practice and a long waiting list used to advise parents of babies with eczema that while they were waiting to get on his schedule, they should simply stop microwaving the baby formula. By the time an appointment became available several months later, the eczema would usually have cleared up just from that one change.

**Milk from plants, not cows.** Cow's milk was designed to turn a baby calf into a half-ton cow. The protein and fat molecules are too big for humans to digest well. Goat's milk is much better for humans because goats are closer in size to humans.

Better yet, use all the wonderful plant-based milks now on the market, made from coconut, almonds, rice, whole grains, and soy. (As for the rumors that soy is dangerous: a billion Chinese and Japanese live on soy and are much healthier than we are. They eat traditionally prepared soy foods, though. I would avoid highly processed soy foods. Americans can't seem to resist monkeying with perfectly good traditional foods.)

Probably the healthiest of all is hemp milk, and no, it won't get you high—it's from a different type of hemp plant. It's a good source of protein and high quality essential fatty acids. You can make your own almond milk and hemp milk in a Vita-Mix.

**If you eat meat, make sure it's grass-fed and grass-finished.** Meat sold in stores is generally not as healthy as meat was 100 years ago, let alone the meat from cave-man days. In fact, it's *anti*-healthy. That's because of the essential fatty acid profile. Wild game has a healthy blend of fatty acids. But the grains fed to animals in modern factory farms transform the fatty acids so they're *un*healthy. That's why there are so many health risks from eating meat, like the well-known connection between eating red meat and developing colon cancer.

Livestock are meant to graze on *grass,* which is why you'll see "grass-fed" blazoned on meats at organic supermarkets. Better yet, try to find grass-*finished* meat, otherwise the animals were fattened up with grains towards the end, which can undo all the benefits of grass-*feeding*.

You'll also need to get organic and hormone/antibiotic-free meat, because antibiotics in the meat breed antibiotic-resistant bacteria and the hormones could contribute to cancer and hormone disruption. You know what gets me upset? Six-year-old girls in my practice developing breast buds and pubic hair. The connection was made years ago between early puberty and hormones in meat.

**Safe sweets.** The sugar substitutes aspartame (Nutrasweet) and sucralose (Splenda) are highly toxic chemicals which never should have been approved for food use. For the whole story about aspartame, read *Excitotoxins: The Taste That Kills* by Russell Blaylock, MD. For sucralose, see **www.greenmedinfo.com/toxic-ingredient/sucralose**. If anything, they are worse than sugar itself. There's no point in using them to diet because recent research shows that they actually stimulate the appetite.

Fortunately, there are safe sugar substitutes now available. Stevia, a natural sweetener made from a plant, is much sweeter than sugar. You only need a few drops of the liquid. Sometimes, though, you (or your kids) want that sugar-crystal look-and-feel. Xylitol, a sweetener made from birch bark, is available for example as Xyla brand, which claims that it "looks, tastes, cooks and bakes like sugar." You know what? It's true. Unlike white sugar, stevia and xylitol will not cause a blood sugar rush followed by an energy crash.

**Eat your SEA vegetables,** rich in the dozens of trace minerals that our bodies need. Many metabolic processes in our body won't work if just one mineral is missing, even in tiny amounts. That's because our ancestors climbed out of the sea, and our body wants that sea environment inside. Sound complicated? Keep it simple—eat sea vegetables. Start with nori, the crispy-salty black wrapping around sushi. It's fabulous by itself as a snack. You can find it in stores like Trader Joe's and Whole Foods (where it's called Sea Tangle). Kids love it.

Next, get nori in sheets (be sure to get the pre-roasted kind because the plain stuff is just plain dull). You'll find it in the Japanese section of your natural grocery, or in a Japanese grocery store if you're lucky enough to have one nearby. Fold a sheet in half and put your sandwich filling in it—tofu salad, chicken salad, hummus and veggies, just about anything but PB&J. Once you've made friends with nori, it's an easy hop to enjoying other sea vegetables. Your body will thank you.

**Grow your own organic vegetables or join a CSA (Community Supported Agriculture) program.** Even in a small backyard plot, you can grow so many vegetables that you won't be able to eat them all. It's a great way to involve kids—kids are much more likely to eat vegetables if they've helped grow them and prepare them. You can learn more from the PBS show *Garden Girl,* now immortalized at **www.Garden GirlTV.com.**

By eating vegetables right after they're picked, you maximize the vitamins. In supermarket vegetables, the vitamin content declines with each day they're trucked across the country, displayed in the store, and neglected in your refrigerator. If you don't believe there's a difference, try eating sweet corn right when it's picked. You don't even need to cook it. The sugar content starts to turn to starch as soon as its picked, so you'll really taste a difference between fresh-picked and store-bought.

As for minerals, you need good mineral rich compost to get the best quality veggies. One study on the mineral content of organic vegetables *purportedly* showed that it was no better than commercial vegetables—but then it turned out that commercial vegetables had been used to compost the organic ones, so they weren't adding anything to the soil. Minerals don't appear out of thin air. You need mineral-rich compost to grow mineral-rich vegetables.

If you don't have access to a small plot of land, consider window-sill gardening, at least for herbs and tomatoes. The website **www.Garden GirlTV.com** teaches you how to set up a whole garden indoors. Check out Britta Riley's TED talk on YouTube, "A Garden In My Apartment." She not only created an indoor garden from recycled materials, she began an international movement of thousands of people sharing ideas and information for energy-efficient hydroponic gardening.

Look for a nearby CSA where you can buy a share in a farm which then typically delivers a big box of fresh vegetables once a week to a location near your house. Sometimes they let you go to the farm and pick your own—a great experience for kids. Find out CSA locations at www.localharvest.org. You'll also be supporting your local farmer, who can make a better living by bypassing the middleman.

**Buy organic/local-grown or fairly traded.** When you do need to shop in a store, look for locally grown or locally made organic foods. You will be supporting the health of your local economy and you'll get better quality food if it's made fresh.

You'll probably need to buy some foods from overseas, like chocolate and coffee (two of my four basic food groups!). Please look for "fairly traded" on the label. That means they were grown by co-ops of local farmers, not a multinational corporation which pays the farmers pennies on the dollar. These local farmers typically commit to growing organically because they see how sick their families get when they use pesticides. Did you know that pesticides banned in the US are exported to other countries and then come back to us on the fruits and other foods we import from those countries? It's harmful for the farmers, for the ecosystem, and for our own health.

Supporting fair trade means reaching a hand across the ocean to support the people growing your food, plus it creates a healthier ecosystem and healthier food for you.

Speaking of shopping local, please support your local independent health food store, if you have one. It's most likely a labor of love for the owners (I can say this because I used to own one), and the staff are generally more knowledgeable than in shopping mall vitamin stores. Local health food stores are usually a community hub and networking center as well as a great source of information, and you will benefit many times over by supporting such a store. Shopping local for all your needs (like your local farmers' market and bookstores) keeps your money circulating in your community and helps build a thriving local economy.

**Avoid food containing GMOs,** the genetically-modified organisms which are now being found to cause food sensitivities. Ever wonder why so many people have to avoid gluten and why so many kids are allergic to peanuts that they had to be banned in schools? When we were growing up, everybody ate everything and nobody had a problem with it.

Leaky gut syndrome lets food particles into your bloodstream where your immune system reacts to them as if they were foreign invaders. Apparently GMO foods both contribute to leaky gut and create particles that act like allergens. But the US doesn't require GMO labeling as other countries do. The solution? Sign the petition at **JustLabelIt.org**, and buy the organic version of the worst offenders: soy, corn, sugar, milk, and cottonseed and canola oil. Yes, these are everywhere in our food supply. Another reason to buy organic.

### Resources for Healthy Cooking

There are many, many wonderful cookbooks for healthy cuisine, and your local health food store should have a good selection. Here are a few less obvious ones. *Feeding the Whole Family* by Cynthia Lair includes ideas for preparing healthy foods for infants and picky eaters. One unique feature: each recipe tells how to adapt it for babies.

If you would like to be inspired by a totally gorgeous book that makes you want to cook natural foods, check out the really delicious healthy recipes in Heidi Swanson's *Super Natural Every Day.*

*If the Buddha Came to Dinner,* would you feed him frozen microwaved TV dinners? And if not, why are you feeding yourself that way? Being more conscious of how you eat makes it easy to eat healthy—because it's what your body actually wants, if you just pay attention. Plus this book by Schatz and Shaiman has wonderful recipes from two healthy traditional cuisines—Japanese and Middle Eastern.

But maybe you have a mental block because you don't know the first thing about cooking for yourself, like many Americans who never learned from their mothers. If so, check out *The Kitchen Counter Cooking School Book* by Kathleen Finn. You'll laugh, maybe you'll cry, and you'll learn how to replace packaged, processed food with the healthier homemade version and save money at the same time.

## Reference Books for Holistic Nutrition

There are many different approaches to healthy eating, many of which contradict each other. Have you noticed? Are you confused?

What I've found after 40 years in this field is that different people respond well to different diets, and that radically different diets can be healthy. One of my customers cured her breast cancer with a raw foods diet—and another one cured hers with macrobiotic foods, which are almost entirely cooked.

One explanation is genetic: for example, the *Eat Right For Your Type* books by Dr. Peter D'Adamo asserts that each blood type needs a different diet. I hear the skeptics snorting at this point, but the fact is that many people I know feel better (and have more energy and lose weight effortlessly) when they follow his recommendations.

But some people don't. So then there are the raw food folks who say that all the life energy in food is destroyed by cooking, as well as the macrobiotics who cook everything because it breaks down the cellulose and makes the nutrients available. Macrobiotics don't tend to use a lot of herbs and spices, but the Ayurvedic cuisine of India uses a sophisticated palette of spices that also double as medicine. Meanwhile, the Paleo diet books will tell you to eat like cave people, with wild game and no grains. It's enough to make you give up and head for the Coke and pizza.

Let's see what these natural approaches to eating tend to *agree* on.

- Fresh fruits and vegetables, organic and local grown if possible.
- Food that looks like it came right out of the ground or the ocean or off the tree. Nothing with labels—at least no labels with chemical-sounding ingredients.
- Whole grains, if you want to eat grains; many people feel better by avoiding gluten (in wheat, rye, barley, and lots of processed foods).
- Meat which is organic, hormone- and antibiotic-free, grass-fed, and in smaller quantities than in our SAD (Standard American Diet).
- Fish from cold water (for good essential fatty acids) and small (low on the food chain, lower in toxins). Definitely not farmed fish, which tends to lack nutrients and contain antibiotics.

∾  High quality oils (virgin organic olive oil and reliable sources of essential fatty acids and maybe ghee/clarified butter).

See? There actually *is* a lot of consensus. And in terms of raw foods versus cooked, a lot of us follow our natural instincts and eat more food raw in the hot weather and cooked when it's cold.

So I would like to encourage you to experiment. Maybe try one new type of food each week. Or maybe go cold turkey and get the positive reinforcement of feeling much better from a radical change. You could begin with a pantry and refrigerator purge of packaged foods, harmful oils, and anything with sugar.

I'm going to make a major pitch here for cooking for yourself and your family (and that means stove, oven, or Vita-Mix not microwave). Food carries consciousness. It can either carry the love you feel for your body and your kids' bodies, or it could carry the cranky mood of an underpaid fast food worker. I know it takes time to prepare your own food. If you have kids, it may seem impossible. Get the kids to help you. The more naturally they eat, the more calm and cooperative they will be. Kids are more likely to eat food they have helped to prepare.

Here are a few cookbooks which advocate a particular approach to eating. Start with the approach that appeals to you and have fun experimenting.

*The Engine 2 Diet* by Rip Esselstyn reflects my own personal preference for a plant-based diet, including only plant proteins from beans, nuts, seeds, and whole grains. Rip, a triathlete and firefighter, transformed the health of his whole firehouse when they did a collective experiment with a plant-based diet based on research by Rip's father, Dr. Caldwell Esselstyn. It also reflects the experience of many of my fellow marathoners and triathletes that we feel better on a non-dairy vegetarian diet. However, I also know people who report feeling weak without animal protein, and for them there are lots of cookbooks following "oldways" traditions like Chinese, Japanese, and Mediterranean, in which meat appears as a condiment.

For those who feel drawn to eating more meat as well as dairy products, consider *Real Food: What to Eat and Why* by Nina Planck, and *Nourishing Traditions* by Sally Fallon. Their "traditional foods" approach is based on the research of Weston Price, a dentist who traveled the world in the 1930s comparing the teeth (and overall health) of traditional peoples with those of "civilized societies." When canned and processed foods arrived in places like Fiji, the chronic diseases of civilization came too, including tooth decay and crowded dental arches. Weston Price researched what traditional diets had in common all over the world and the result is reflected in these books. He recommends meat and milk—but only raw and preferably fermented milk, which is hard for most Americans to come by.

In terms of raw versus cooked food, you could try the seasonal approach in *Staying Healthy with the Seasons* by Elson Haas, MD and *Healing with Whole Foods: Asian Traditions and Modern Nutrition* by Paul Pitchford, which uses the "five season" approach of Traditional Chinese Medicine.

### THE TOXIC TOMATO

I had a little vegetarian cafe in my health food store with seating for eight people. One day a mother brought her college-student daughter in for lunch, clearly in some attempt to patch up their relationship.

The daughter interrogated me about the ingredients in the felafel sandwich on a whole wheat pita (organic whole wheat and chickpeas, no dairy in the tahini dressing, and so forth). It seemed to pass muster but then after one bite she started screaming. It had a tomato in it, and believing nightshade vegetables to be toxic, she was sure she had been poisoned!

Needless to say, this ruined the lunch, and I wished I could tell her that sometimes the *feeling* behind the food is more important than the ingredient list!

# SIMPLE SUGGESTIONS
# FOR DAILY SUPPLEMENTS

I love the concept of getting all the nutrients we need from food. But it's just that—a nice *idea*.

Our ancestors were able to do it, up until the last century. Actually, let's get specific: up until World War II. What happened then? "Better living through chemistry." The chemical industry polluted our environment with thousands of chemicals which we did not evolve to deal with. Most have never been tested for safety, and none have been tested for safety in combination with other chemicals. We're all the guinea pigs.

Agribusiness also developed after World War II: huge farms growing only one crop (and therefore more susceptible to insects, hence the need for pesticides) with chemical fertilizers, which only replace a couple of the minerals the plants need. It's sort of like "enriched" bread with just a few synthetic vitamins added back in to replace the many nutrients lost in milling. For more about this, read the section on potato farming in Michael Pollan's *The Botany of Desire*. Read it—and weep. The potato farmers won't eat their own commercially-grown potatoes; they keep a kitchen garden by the back porch for potatoes grown the old-fashioned way.

Our conventional produce also lacks vitamins because it's been trucked across the country, losing vitamins along the way, and losing more while it sits in the store and then sits in your refrigerator. Plus factory farming has depleted the minerals in our soil, so our vegetables end up without the minerals they are supposed to have.

We have a greater *need* for nutrients than ever before because our bodies are more challenged than ever—dealing not only with the proliferation of chemicals, but also with many other nutrient-depleting factors like electromagnetic fields, fluorescent lights, and stress. So we need *more* nutrients than our pre-World War II ancestors, while we're getting much *less*.

Do you think of organic foods as a frivolous expense, a sort of "unnatural" indulgence for health nuts? Think again. Your great-grandparents ate only organic—because that's all there was. They also ate from their own gardens or local truck farms. They spent a lot more time outside in the fresh aid and sunshine than we do. They got more physical exercise because physical labor was much more a part of life. To see a smart and savvy analysis of why organic is more expensive (and shouldn't be), go to YouTube for the TED talk of Robyn O'Brien, a food industry analyst turned food activist.

We're dealing with a really unhealthy lifestyle here, and supplements are just a way to bring us up to baseline. So here are my bottom-line recommendations, for the best results with the least number of pills.

Before I start, let me make the pitch for natural rather than synthetic vitamins. Natural vitamins are more expensive and they're worth it because the body recognizes them and can use them more effectively. When you see a study that *purports* to prove that vitamins don't work, or are toxic, the vitamins used in the study were synthetic. Synthetic vitamins also tend to be isolated, whereas natural vitamins occur in groups. (I'm thinking of vitamin E, which is a blend of tocopherols, and the carotenes, of which beta carotene is just a single element.) Yes, taking just one synthetic vitamin out of a group *can* be harmful because it throws the levels of all the others out of whack. Vitamins aren't isolated in nature, and they shouldn't be in your supplements either.

Finally, natural supplements use better quality source ingredients which tend to be better absorbed in the body. Please don't shortchange yourself with a cheap synthetic vitamin. Get a good natural brand. Your health is worth it.

These recommendations are likely to be higher than the RDAs, because the RDAs are only meant to prevent deficiency diseases (is preventing scurvy your only concern here?) and in any case they only apply to healthy people. You need more than the RDA if you have a chronic illness, pain or other medical condition, if you exercise or are under stress, if you are very young, elderly, pregnant or nursing. I hope you're not under stress, but I do hope you are exercising!

As for the cost, if you spend more on organic food and supplements, you'll more than make it up with health care savings. Fewer colds, fewer co-pays, less time lost from work. Healthy food is cheap compared to medical care.

Here's one more thing to consider, before you head for your local health food store to get some excellent quality nutritional supplements. You could get your supplemental nutrients in *food-grown* form which will seem relatively low-potency on the label, but they will absorb well because your body will recognize them as food. Or you can get a good-quality natural brand of vitamins *added to a base of food*, which will have higher amounts on the label. You might have more confidence in this type, such as Rainbow Light brand. Personally I like the food-*grown* supplements like the MegaFoods brand.

So here's my bottom line for people who want a simple, manageable routine. These are starting suggestions. If you have an excellent whole-organic-foods diet, you'll need less; if you're under extra stress or have other nutrient-depleting factors, you'll need more. For additional information and research studies, see the Notes section.

### For a Healthy Young Adult, Age 16 to 39

**A good multivitamin,** for example Megafoods for a food-grown brand; Rainbow Light for a higher-potency brand with an excellent quality food base; Synergy Basic by NSI for a cost-effective synthetic option. Look for 400mcg of folate plus mixed carotenoids. If you don't like swallowing pills, get a good powdered form like All-One and add it to a smoothie.

**Vitamin C:** several grams (several thousand milligrams). I like raspberry Emergen-C, which makes a fizzy drink. When you're sick, you may need 1000 milligrams an hour (in buffered form so it's easier on the stomach). Keep taking it until you get diarrhea (the bowel tolerance test), then back off. Your body will use up much more than you expect.

**Vitamin D3:** 2,000 to 5,000 IU. 2,000 IU is the maintenance dose once you've gotten your blood level up to at least 50 (see Notes for information about testing and contraindications). Most people have much lower blood level: take 5,000 IU a day for three months and then retest. Ideally you'll get your D from sunshine during the summer months: at least half an hour a day in full sun, then you don't need the supplement.

**Fish oil (Omega 3):** 1000 mg. Nordic Naturals is an excellent brand. Women should take their Nordic Natural for Women, men their Ultimate Omega. If you want to use a different brand, make sure it is molecularly distilled, which means any mercury has been distilled out of it, and as a side benefit it's unlikely to cause "fishy burps." There's new evidence that plant-based essential fatty acids are even better, such as Barlean's Ultimate Omega Swirl. The version for women's hormone balancing is Chocolate Raspberry and honestly, it's good enough to eat by the spoonful right out of the bottle, as I am wont to do. On the other hand, many people prefer Fermented Cod Liver Oil by Green Pastures, prepared the traditional way for best absorption of the nutrients.

**A good probiotic** with *billions* (not hundreds of millions) of organisms per capsule, such as Jarro-Dophilus or MegaFood's MegaFlora.

**Calcium and magnesium:** 250 to 500 mg calcium and at least as much magnesium. (The amount you need varies widely depending on your food and exercise; see the Osteoporosis section on page 120.) Avoid calcium *carbonate,* which is poorly absorbed, contributing to hardening of the arteries, "gravel" in the joints, and kidney stones. Well-absorbed forms include citrates and orotates, actually anything that ends in "–ate" except carbonate. Pioneer Calcium Magnesium Bone Protein and Trace

Mineral Complex is an unusually good formula, with added trace minerals and protein needed for strong bones.

**A green food powder** (like spirulina, chlorella or blue-green algae mixed with powdered vegetables) unless you are really, really good about eating a *lot* of green vegetables. You can add these powders to smoothies. Start small (1/4 to 1/2 tsp) and gradually increase. They won't change the flavor much but they will turn your fruit smoothie a startling blue-green.

**Vitamin B12** if you don't eat animal foods: 10 micrograms a day or 2000 once a week. B12 is only needed in tiny amounts, but it's really important. Vegans (people who eat no animal foods) tend to be low in B12, leading to anemia and fatigue and, worst case scenario, a heart attack or stroke. B12 is not absorbed well through the stomach, so you need a form that dissolves in the mouth like Jarrow's Methyl-B12.

## Adjustments for Older Adults

- ∾ **A multi for older people** such as MegaFoods "Over 40" products, or Rainbow Light Active Senior, or NSI's Synergy Basic 3.
- ∾ **Fish oil:** increase to 2000 mg (see notes if you are on coumadin).
- ∾ **CoQ10** as Ubiquinol, 60 mg (for heart health and more energy).
- ∾ **Vitamin K2** such as Jarrow MK7, for strong bones, arteries, and blood clotting (coordinate with your doctor if on blood thinners).
- ∾ **A supplement for your eyes,** such as Gaia's Vision Enhancement.

## Adjustments for Children

- ∾ **A children's multi** such as MegaFoods Kids' or Rainbow Light Kids One (hypoallergenics); kids in my practice also like Nordic Naturals Nordic Berries.
- ∾ **An age-appropriate probiotic,** perhaps the most important supplement to keep your child from getting sick, such as

MegaFoods Kids-N-Us MegaFlora. Babies and toddlers need different strains of beneficial bacteria, and Renew Life FloraBaby is a big favorite among the moms in my practice.

∾ **Fish oils** such as Nordic Naturals ProDHA, 2 caps a day. (If they're too small to swallow capsules, prick the caps, add to juice.). DHA is most important for brain development. If the child suffers from mood or behavior problems, substitute Nordic Naturals ProEPA.

∾ **Vitamin D3**, 400 IU, or more if your child has no sun exposure.

### Books for Healing Chronic Conditions with Healthy Food and Supplements

The previous section was about a basic daily regimen. If you're actually dealing with a chronic illness, though, you'll need additional specialized supplements. I would follow these recommendations *in addition to* professional care from a functional medicine doctor, naturopath, and/or a homeopath (see pages 237–240).

If you can't afford professional holistic care or can't find an appropriate holistic doctor in your area, try following the recommendations in these books/websites in addition to *conventional* medical care. Don't try to treat a chronic illness on your own.

None of these books cover homeopathic medicines for *chronic* conditions because they have to be tailored to you like a custom-fitted suit, and you just can't do that for yourself. Homeopathy is especially effective for *stress*-related chronic illnesses.

*Prescription for Natural Cures* by James F. Balch, MD, Mark Stengler, NMD, and Robin Young Balch, ND is the updated version of the classic *Prescription for Nutritional Healing.* Search hundreds of health conditions for recommendations as to supplements, herbs, homeopathics, and dietary changes.

*UltraMetabolism, UltraPrevention, The UltraMind Solution, The Blood Sugar Solution* and other books by Dr. Mark Hyman. He has done an amazing job of compiling excellent holistic information in very readable form, complete with meal plans, recipes, and supplement suggestions. You can also find his articles at **www.DrHyman.com.**

*From Fatigued to Fantastic, Beat Sugar Addiction Now, Pain Free 1-2-3,* and *Real Cause, Real Cure* by Dr. Jacob Teitelbaum address chronic fatigue, fibromyalgia, chronic pain, and other health problems which can only be cured with natural food and supplements.

*Radical Medicine* by Dr. Louise L. Williams explains how to go to the root of disease, providing effective traditional holistic solutions to ultra-modern health problems.

*Why Do I Still Have Thyroid Symptoms When My Lab Tests Are Normal?* by Dr. Darit Kharrazian is the best explanation I've found of the complex reasons for hypothyroidism. You'll need to find a naturopathic doctor trained in his method, but at least you'll have good understanding.

## Websites for Chronic Health Problems

**www.GreenMedInfo.com** has "the world's largest evidence-based, open source, natural medicine database" citing research from mainstream medical and scientific journals in a database of almost 20,000 articles. This site is a treasure trove of reliable information about holistic health care, backed by science, yet easily understandable by the average reader.

**www.Orthomolecular.org** provides the free Orthomolecular Medicine News Service, which is excellent both for the vitamins and supplements it recommends, and also for its well-documented rebuttals to the vitamin-bashing in the media (which is based on twisted statistics, as you'll learn on this site). Issues from before 2007 are archived at **www.Doctor Yourself.com** and are still timely. This latter site also highlights the books of Dr. Andrew Saul such as *Doctor Yourself: Natural Medicine That Works* (and by "natural medicine" he means high-potency supplements). He also has a book that seems unique among those we recommend here: *Hospitals and Health,* about taking charge of your health (your food, your vitamins, your toxic exposure) while in the hospital.

**www.KnowledgeofHealth.com** features the informative blogs, and **www. NaturalHealthLibrarian.com** features the books, of "nutrition physician" Dr. Bill Sardi. His best-known book is *Downsizing Your Body,* about weight loss, plus he has written many others on a wide variety of health conditions, and about the benefits—or dangers—of specific supplements.

**www.DrMercola.com and www.NaturalNews.com** have important information about natural alternatives to drugs, from Dr. Mercola and "Health Ranger" Mike Adams respectively. These people are really courageous. Their own articles are generally well grounded. You just need to think for yourself about information posted by "citizen journalists" on NaturalNews.com, and information about products for sale on DrMercola.com—much of the info is good, some of it is questionable.

### Websites for Healthy Food and Holistic Nutrition

There is some overlap here: the previous sites focused on healing specific disease conditions, whereas the following sites provide all-around information for a healthy lifestyle, and of course they tend to cover some of the same ground.

**www.HappyHealthyLongLife.com** is "a medical librarian's adventures in evidence-based living." This anonymous librarian reviews new books, research studies, products, and recipes after testing them out on herself. The writing is clear, colorful, and a joy to read. Her posts are well organized by topic, and she has dozens of interesting topics to explore. Have fun cruising around this website.

**www.HealthyGirlsKitchen.blogspot.com** has great vegan recipes including 40 recipes for green smoothies, many of them "kid-tested."

**www.YourHealthWorks.com** includes information about healthy food, a healthy home, and natural healing for lots of conditions.

**www.101Cookbooks.com** is the website of Heidi Swanson, whose *Super Natural Every Day* I recommended as an absolutely gorgeous and inspiring cookbook. Her website has some really practical features in addition to great recipes. For example, under Recipes, check out "A few favorite oils," "A few favorite sweeteners" and "A few favorite grains." Everything I would have said on these topics, she says better. While you're there, download her recipe for Magic Sauce, an intensely flavored sauce with fresh herbs. There are infinite possible variations depending on what flavors you like, and infinite ways to use it. This one sauce can make everything taste better. Gone are the days of bland and heavy natural foods.

**www.CookusInterruptus.com** is totally fun. Its short videos show you "how to cook fresh local organic whole foods despite life's interruptions." The recipes are simple and tasty, with gluten-free options, suggestions for kids, and tips for finding local foods. Plus the goofy sense of humor makes the videos easy to watch. Videos of basic cooking techniques are listed under *How to Boil Water*. See what I mean about goofy humor?

### Books and Websites for Kids' Health

**Nutrition and Your Child's Soul** by Dolev Gilmore covers many aspects of children's health, not just nutrition, with wit and wisdom and a heartfelt plea for the health of your child.

**www.NourishMD.com** is a website run by a pediatrician and a holistic nutritionist, both moms. Their website focuses on healthy food and supplements and how to get kids to eat them or take them.

**www.FoodForKidsHealth.com** features "solutions for picky eaters: make your kids smarter, healthier and better behaved" plus great information on natural baby formula, food allergies, foods to enhance fertility, and much more.

**www.KellyDorfman.com** is the website of Kelly Dorfman, a holistic nutritionist specializing in healing kids with learning and behavior disorders by changing their diets and adding a few special supplements. She has lots of informative articles and a blog that's both educational and entertaining. This woman is one of the smartest, savviest people I've met, and her website is definitely worth checking out along with her book, *What's Eating Your Child?*

# HEALTHY EMOTIONAL EXPRESSION

As a homeopath, I see many examples of chronic physical ailments brought about by suppressed emotions. You know the little jiggler valve on top of a pressure cooker? Suppressed emotions are the pressure building up in the pressure cooker . . . the pressure has to find a way out, and if the emotions are not voiced, then the body may "speak" through physical symptoms.

You would be surprised how often physical symptoms mirror the language of the emotions. Clients will use the same words to describe a crushing headache and being crushed by a relationship . . . or an angry rash while they try to deny feeling anger at their spouse . . . or feeling invaded by intrusive in-laws while their immune system is being invaded by pathogens. Part of our healing paradigm in homeopathy is that the physical symptom cannot heal, in a deep and lasting way, until any underlying emotional trauma is resolved.

So I encourage my clients to find ways to express themselves in a calm, clear way that invites negotiation rather than shutting down communication. There are hundreds of wonderful books, therapies, approaches, and experts. The following are personal favorites or ones that have been life-transforming for my clients.

As a longtime meditator, I especially appreciate books that use the tools of meditation and spirituality to help lift us up from psychological suffering, for example:

∞ *The Mindful Way through Depression: Freeing Yourself from Chronic Unhappiness* by Williams, Teasale, Kabat-Zinn, and Segal.

∞ *Coming to Our Senses: Healing Ourselves and the World through Mindfulness* by Jon Kabat-Zinn.

∞ *The Mindful Path to Self-Compassion* by Christopher Germer.

### Finding Ways to Communicate Difficult Emotions Honestly and Effectively

*The Dance of Anger* by Harriet Goldhor Lerner: This classic book is a perpetual favorite among my clients (and required reading for those who need Staphysagria, a homeopathic medicine for chronic illness due to suppressed anger). It teaches people that it's okay to be angry, that everyone gets angry at some point, and that you don't have to be *right* to be angry. It's enough that you simply feel angry.

Then it coaches you on effective ways to express the anger, like speaking up when you first start to notice that you're getting irritated instead of putting it off until you have a volcanic eruption. Another technique is to express yourself in terms of "When you do that, I feel this" (which can't be argued with) rather than "You shouldn't do that," which sounds scolding and judgmental.

*Difficult Conversations* by Stone, Patton and Heen, members of the Harvard Negotiation Project: Here are a couple of my favorite tips from this book about how to have a conversation you dread. Instead of trying to assign blame, ask each person how they *contributed* to the problem at hand, with the idea that everyone contributes something when things have gone awry. Also, try to separate *intent* from *impact*: someone's actions may have had a painful effect on you, but most likely the other person did not *intend* to hurt you.

There's so much more wisdom in both of these books, I feel that everyone would benefit from them.

## Emotional Health for Kids

*How to Talk So Kids Will Listen and Listen So Kids Will Talk* by Adele Faber and Elaine Mazlich is a perennial favorite among my clients. (Honestly, though, some kids in my practice are so wild that talking won't work and they really do need natural healing interventions first.) *The Blessing of a Skinned Knee* by Wendy Vogel is full of sage advice drawing on Jewish wisdom stories. A psychotherapist colleague recommends the free online course called "Raising Happiness" from Dr. Christine Carter, a sociologist at UC Berkeley. She has also written a book of the same title. **www.RaisingHappiness.com.**

## The Physical Basis for Emotional Health

Sometimes what we perceive as depression or anxiety is actually a physical problem — a lack of nutrients, an improper balance of essential fatty acids (because our brains and nervous system are largely made of fats), or a toxic load of heavy metals. Dr. Mark Hyman's *The UltraMind Solution: The Simple Way to Defeat Depression, Overcome Anxiety, and Sharpen Your Mind* will tell you what supplements to take and what foods to eat. He also explains the science behind his suggestions.

# MENTAL CLARITY

Good nutrition helps our brains function well throughout the lifespan, from kids with ADHD to aging baby boomers. The brain needs so many special nutrients that I cannot do the topic justice here. Instead I'll refer you to Dr. Mark Hyman's *UltraMind Solution*; Dr. Daniel Amen's series on the brain; and the works of my brilliant colleague, Dr. Charles Krebs. Specific nutrients for children are addressed in Kelly Dorfman's *What's Eating Your Child?*

At the Lydian Center for Innovative Medicine, where I work with brain experts including chiropractors, neuroacupressure practitioners, and a Brain Gym practitioner, we have a motto: The brain needs movement to grow. My colleagues recommend Brain Gym for a wide variety of situations, from children with learning disabilities to stroke victims.

Brain Gym helps to increase the connection among parts of the brain and even to develop alternative pathways when a part of the brain has been damaged by an accident or stroke. It's a series of exercises that kids enjoy and anyone can do. They are deceptively simple; neurophysiologist Dr. Carla Hannaford explains how they stimulate brain connections in her *Smart Moves: Why Learning Is Not All in Your Head*. You can learn how to do them from Dr. Paul Dennison's *Brain Gym, Teachers' Edition;* more information at **www.BrainGym.org**.

# SUPPORT YOUR BODY'S
# HEALING ENERGY

The body's own natural healing energy is called *chi* in Traditional Chinese Medicine and the Vital Force in homeopathy. It's what animates the body, the life force that moves it, the spirit that transforms it from what would otherwise be just a hunk of inanimate flesh.

I tried to explain this concept to my father the doctor. He thought about it for a while. "You know," he said, "you can take two elderly ladies with venous ulcers" (the hard-to-heal ulcers in the legs of frail elderly people). "One lady is still married, lives near her grandchildren, is active in her church, and enjoys working in her garden. The other one is widowed, isolated, depressed, never goes out, never sees anyone. The first one will get better and the second one will not."

"That's it, dad!" I said. "The first lady has a strong Vital Force, that's why her body is able to heal. Did they teach you that concept in medical school?"

"No," my dad said, "but any doctor who's been in practice for a while is familiar with it." So the body's healing energy is *explicitly* addressed in the energy-based healing modalities like acupuncture and homeopathy, while it's a silent partner in mainstream Western medicine.

If your Vital Force is weak, here are some ways you can strengthen it. My personal favorite—and something I recommend to everyone—is the **Donna Eden Five-Minute Daily Energy Routine.** It really does take just five minutes (well, maybe 10 because you'll enjoy it so much you'll want to linger over it).

You can see energy healer Karen Semmelman explain it and demonstrate it on my YouTube channel, GreenHealingTV. Look for the Energy episodes. Or you can do a search on YouTube and see energy queen Donna Eden demonstrate it herself.

**Other energy-based exercises** such as yoga, Tai Chi, Qi Gong, aikido, and the Tibetan Five Rites can strengthen your healing energy. I find the complex movements of Tai Chi hard to follow, but I find the simpler patterns of Qi Gong easy and just as effective.

The Tibetan Five Rites, also easy, are described in Peter Kelder's *The Fountain of Youth*, or search YouTube for demonstration videos. Many people have found that these simple exercises restore youthfulness.

**Deep breathing** of fresh pure air will bring *prana* (life-energy) into your system. Alternate nostril breathing is especially effective:

- Touch the root of your nose with your index and middle fingers to hold your hand steady.
- Use your thumb to open and close one nostril.
- Use your ring and pinkie fingers for the other one.
- Breathe in one side (holding the opposite nostril closed).
- Hold for a few seconds, both nostrils closed.
- Breathe out the opposite side.
- Always breathe in on the same side you just breathed out.
- Only have one nostril open at a time while breathing.

Confusing? It's much simpler to do than to describe, and there are lots of demo videos on YouTube. Try it out on your kid when she's getting more and more wound up. Naturopathic doctor Amy Rothenberg, who gets great results treating hyperactive kids with homeopathy, says it can even calm down these kids!

Speaking of breathing fresh pure air . . .

# GET STRENGTH FROM NATURE

Human beings need to stay connected with the energy of the earth. You know how different you feel walking in the woods, or barefoot in the grass, or ankle deep in the ocean with wet sand underfoot? If you don't, you need to get out more! We receive energy from the earth and from having green growing things around us. *Your Brain on Nature* by doctors Selhub and Logan documents the positive effects of nature on your brain, undoing the damaging effects of our wired technology.

If you're a city-dweller, here are a few things you can do.

**Get an Earthing Mat** from www.Earthing.net. Mine has made a huge difference for me. It helps to balance out the energy drain from spending hours on the computer. If you want to know the science behind it, get *Earthing: The Most Important Health Discovery Ever?* or head on over to their website, **www.Grounded.com,** for a good basic explanation of why this simple product can make such a difference in how you feel.

**Block electromagnetic radiation.** Speaking of all the wonderful positive energy we can absorb from the earth, and how our modern lifestyle blocks us from it, reminds me that we also need to minimize our exposure to electromagnetic fields. We're all swimming in a soup of radiation from cell phone towers, computers, electrical wiring, estimated to be 100 million times stronger than the radiation field that our grandparents were exposed to, and it could be contributing to everything from chronic fatigue to cancer to infertility.

This is such a huge topic, I can only beg you to get Ann Louise Gittleman's *Zapped: Why Your Cell Phone Shouldn't Be Your Alarm Clock and 1,268 Ways to Outsmart the Hazards of Electronic Pollution.* First she'll scare your pants off and then she'll tell you what to do about it.

**Grow a garden.** Plugging in your Earthing mat and protecting yourself from electromagnetic fields are high tech ways of benefiting from the earth's healing energy. But there's nothing like actually getting your hands dirty in a garden. With even a small patch of ground, you can grow your own organic vegetables in a raised-bed garden. (The raised-bed lets you put in good clean dirt, and you don't have to bend over so far.) Learn about urban gardening—including indoor gardening—from "The Garden Girl" and her PBS show at **www.GardenGirlTV.com**.

**Take your child out in nature.** The "No Child Left Inside" movement reflects a new awareness of how important it is for kids to experience nature. Richard Louv coined the term "Nature Deficit Disorder" in his *Last Child in the Woods,* one of my favorites. He cites recent research linking time spent in nature with reduced symptoms for kids diagnosed with ADHD. The Children and Nature Network connects kids, families, and communities to nature "through innovative ideas, evidence-based resources and tools, broad-based collaboration, and support of grassroots leadership." Check out their website for practical tips and research on humans' need for nature: **www.ChildrenandNature.org**.

**www.FreeRangeKids.wordpress.com** This blog is about empowering kids, encouraging them to walk, bike and go out in nature, and overcoming the culture of fear in our society that keeps kids inside. The author, Lenore Skenazy, promotes teaching kids good self-defense techniques and then using common sense in letting them go outside.

She laments something I've noticed in my neighborhood where I grew up: where are all the kids? Safely inside watching TV, I guess. In the old days the neighborhood was teeming with kids riding bikes and playing in each others' yards. Now the kids are inside, and it's lonely.

# THE POWER OF
# MIND-BODY MEDICINE

True, visualizations and positive affirmations are not products you can put on the shelf of your natural medicine cabinet. But they are natural, they're free, they're safe, and their effectiveness is well documented with research studies in hospitals all over the country.

Dr. Herbert Benson at Harvard Medical School was the pioneer way back in the '70s, documenting the benefits of the Relaxation Response not only for stress reduction but also for high blood pressure, PMS, and many other physical conditions. And for those of you who might feel silly chanting a mantra, he devised a secular version of Transcendental Meditation: you just have to breathe deeply and silently chant "one" for 15 to 20 minutes. Dr. Benson's technique is described—along with extensive research to document it—in *The Relaxation Response*. There are many CDs based on the Relaxation Response available online.

Dr. Jon Kabat-Zinn's Mindfulness-Based Stress Reduction program, similarly based on meditation as well as yoga, has helped tens of thousands of people around the world. Like the Relaxation Response, it reduces stress and anxiety, which skeptics might attribute to the placebo effect. But how can the placebo effect explain his program's effect on *physical* symptoms like psoriasis, immune response, and pain that does not respond to conventional painkillers?

Dr. Kabat-Zinn's books include *Mindfulness for Beginners* and *Wherever You Go, There You Are*. His CDs include *Guided Mindfulness*

*Meditation, Mindfulness Meditation for Pain Relief,* and *The Mindful Way Through Depression.*

Peggy Huddleston's *Prepare for Surgery, Heal Faster* outlines a series of steps to prepare for surgery using mind-body techniques she developed to help people reduce anxiety before surgery. To her surprise, she discovered that it gave physical benefits which could not possibly be explained by the placebo effect — including shorter hospital stays and reduced need for medication (only Tylenol after open heart surgery?!). In brief, her method includes:

- Reducing anxiety by listening to her 20-minute relaxation CD (the immune system responds dramatically in research studies).
- Turning your worries and fears into healing imagery (for example, visualizing a wound healing actually speeds up its healing time).
- Organizing a support group to surround you with love before surgery.
- Using Healing Statements, words spoken during surgery by the anesthesiologist (resulting in 23% to 50% less pain medication, depending on the study).

As the lead author of one of the research studies stated, if a medication got results like this, it would be immediately adopted in every hospital in the US. Her book and CD can also be applied to reducing the side effects of cancer treatment and to healing chronic illnesses such as lupus. Much more information is available at **www.HealFaster.com.**

So what if you "don't believe in all this stuff"? It will still work, according to Huddleston's research. However, if you feel self-conscious doing it, you can have someone else do it for you. Or if your aging parents are recalcitrant, you can do it for them. It's a great way to channel the love and concern you feel for someone going through a health crisis, and to transform the natural fears that come up into visualizing a positive outcome.

What about using this type of mind-body technique for the lumps and bumps you'll be treating with your natural home medicine cabinet? You can visualize pouring your love and healing intent into your herbs and homeopathics. My spiritual teacher, Sri Chinmoy, used to suggest praying for someone, then putting the power of your prayer into the homeopathic medicine you are administering. This is a wonderful way to connect with your loved ones when they are ill, and it will help you to feel engaged and effective rather than feeling powerless.

There are many forms of meditation, and different kinds work for different people. In my own classes (more info at **www.FreeMeditation Boston.org**), I teach heart-center meditation, focusing on the heart center or heart *chakra* as a way to escape from our busy minds and find a source of peace deep inside the core of our being. You might find that a different kind works for you, though, such as a Buddhist style of meditation, which tends to be more psychological and cerebral. You can also find meditative practices for Christians, such as centering prayer, and for Jews, such as reflecting on the daily lessons of Mussar or doing mystical practices based on the Kabbalah.

In my classes I use Sri Chinmoy's *Flute Music for Meditation* and *Aum Ocean Meditation* (which combines restful ocean waves with flute music and the chant of Aum, **www.Heart-Light.com**). For a guided meditation, I recommend Sujantra McKeever's CD *Focus Relax Peace*. My colleagues offer free meditation classes in major cities worldwide, listed at **www.SriChinmoyCentre.org**.

Whatever type of meditation you like, you'll derive great benefits—physical, mental, and spiritual—from practicing it regularly, even for just a few minutes a day. It will help you remain calm and centered, in touch with your higher purpose on earth, and more aware of what you're feeling inside—and that will help you take charge of your own health.

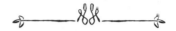

## PART TWO

# DRUG-FREE REMEDIES FOR COMMON AILMENTS

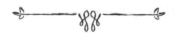

This section covers about 200 common ailments. If you can't find the one you're looking for, check the index — it might be included in a larger category like **First Aid** or **Travel Tips**. Please be sure to read **What's Safe to Treat at Home** first.

For each ailment, there's a **Quick Fix** — a short list of things likely to give you results right away. Most often they are homeopathic remedies because I've found that homeopathy works faster than vitamins and herbs. To get results with homeopathy, read about how to use it in **Section Four**. It's a bit tricky to use at first but you'll get the hang of it.

Vitamins, herbs, and other supplements are necessary, though, even if you can't feel them working right away. These show up in the **Ongoing Support** section for each ailment.

Finally, depending on the condition, there's a **Preventing Recurrence** or **Lifestyle Support** section that gives you the bigger picture of how to improve your health concerning this particular condition.

# WHAT'S SAFE
# TO TREAT AT HOME

This is a guide, not a complete list. Be safe and don't take chances. When in doubt, call your doctor or 9-1-1.

Work with a doctor who knows you are using natural remedies, and who will help you know what's safe and what's not. Doctors may have different guidelines for you based on their own experience or on what they know about your medical history.

Using natural medicines invites you to be more aware of yourself and family members. Being aware of what's normal makes you notice when you're out of sorts. What's normal for your thirst, your digestion, your pee-and-poop system? For women, what's a period typically like? Do you keep track of how often you get them? If your body seems out of whack, it helps to know where you are in your cycle.

How about your kids? How warm does their forehead usually feel? How fast do they typically breathe after a soccer game? If you have a toddler, you could get an otoscope and get used to what your child's eardrums look like when she's well, so you know if they look different when she might be sick. For kids who can't answer your questions yet, it's especially important to be observant of how their body normally functions.

So when you're trying to decide whether to treat something at home, call your doctor, or go to the ER:

**Consider the situation:** Use common sense.

ᕦ If this is a condition for which you would normally call 9-1-1 or take the person to the ER, do that. You can give remedies on the way, or while waiting for the EMTs to arrive.

ᕦ Do not delay seeking conventional medical assistance.

ᕦ Once the person is under the care of the EMTs or hospital, do not give remedies unless the person requests it on the spot, or unless it's your own child (for legal reasons).

ᕦ It's generally not advisable to treat someone else's child with non-conventional methods, even with the best of intentions and even in an emergency, without the express permission of the parents.

**Consider the condition:** Use common sense as to whether it's safe to use homeopathy and delay conventional treatment.

If you have small children, it might be wise to have more detailed information than these general guidelines. Cummings and Ullman's *Everybody's Guide to Homeopathic Medicine* has guidelines specifically related to particular conditions.

Here are some typical signs indicating that you should seek conventional care urgently:

**Difficulty breathing** for any reason including if the person has been stung by a bee or swallowed something that can't be coughed up.

**Rapid breathing** should always be evaluated, keeping in mind that children normally breathe faster than adults, and of course people normally breathe faster after exercise.

**Wheezing:** Moderate or severe wheezing with difficulty breathing.

**Mental state: confusion or lack of awareness** of surroundings in someone normally mentally healthy can indicate a severe infection or other serious condition. Loss of consciousness following a head injury.

**Fevers:** A rectal temp over 100.4° F (38° C) in a child under three months, or a baby with a fever and a bulging soft spot on the top of the head.

ॐ  In others, a fever of 104° F (40° C) especially if other signs of illness.

ॐ  Any fever of more than 102° F (39° C) for more than 3 days.

ॐ  Keep in mind that other signs of illness can be more important in evaluating a fever than the temperature: consider energy level, demeanor, mood, and signs of infection. A non-dangerous fever should be left to do its healing work (see story on page 49)

**Loss of fluids:** Prolonged fever or vomiting and/or diarrhea can lead to **dehydration.** A baby can become dehydrated in only 24 hours, older children and adults in just a couple of days. This could require intravenous fluids in the hospital.

**Seizures:** For example, after a head injury. Febrile seizures (during a fever in a small child) usually last less than 5 minutes and are considered benign, but call for help if they go on longer than 10 minutes.

**Stroke:** according to the National Stroke Association, look for these signs, which would indicate calling 9-1-1 immediately:

ॐ  Sudden numbness or weakness of the face, arm, or leg, especially on one side of the body.

ॐ  Sudden confusion, trouble speaking or understanding.

ॐ  Sudden trouble seeing in one or both eyes.

ॐ  Sudden trouble walking, dizziness, loss of balance or coordination.

ॐ  Sudden, severe headache with no known cause.

**Vomiting:** If severe and prolonged, especially after a head injury.

**Eyes:**

ॐ  Severe eye pain, injury to the eye

ॐ  Chemical or foreign object in the eye

ॐ  Loss of vision

ॐ  If light causes pain in the eye

ॐ  If the pupil is shaped irregularly or does not react to changes in light.

**Bleeding:**
- ∾ Unexplained bleeding from the mouth, nose, or rectum; or bloody urine.
- ∾ Bleeding or fluid from nose or ears following head injury.
- ∾ Bleeding from a cut that won't stop.

**Abdominal pain:** Check for appendicitis by pressing in firmly with a finger in the lower right part of the abdomen and letting go. Pain on releasing your finger ("rebound tenderness") is a strong indicator for appendicitis, which is a serious emergency.

**Kidney pain:** This can indicate a kidney infection, a potentially very serious condition. This is especially likely if the person has recently had a urinary tract infection and now has lower back pain with a high fever. Have the person lean over a chair and tap gently with your fist on the spot where the lowest rib attaches to the spine. Pain at that spot is probably kidney pain, which would indicate a kidney infection and the need for urgent conventional care.

**Animal bites:** If from an unknown (possibly rabid) animal, or if red streaks start leading towards the heart.

**Rare, very dangerous conditions:** Unlikely to happen but you should memorize these symptoms:
- ∾ A child who is leaning forward, drooling, can't swallow or talk, looks like throat is closed up (could be epiglottitis).
- ∾ Stiff neck with headache, fever, pain when the head is bent forward (could be meningitis).

This is by no means a complete list. Be safe. Call your doctor if in doubt.

### A MOM IN A PANIC

"She's got a high fever!" was the panicked message on my voice mail from an anxious mom in my practice. "How high?" I asked when I called back. "99 degrees!" Okay, let's take a deep breath here. 98.6° is normal, so 99° barely registers on the fever scale. A mom's anxiety can be worse for kids than the actual condition. Take a deep breath, breathe with your child, send love from your heart to hers. Sometimes that's the best medicine.

And the best medicine for a fever can be simply a lukewarm sponge bath. Fevers are one of the body's ways of mobilizing white blood cells to fight an infection. Forcing the body not to have a fever (by giving a fever-lowering medicine, whether from the drugstore or the herb garden) can prolong an infectious illness.

My colleague Miranda Castro has a reassuring and informative article on "Fevers and Children" on her website, **www.MirandaCastro.com**. She'll calm you down if you're panicked and give lots of instructions for supporting a child's healing energy during a fever, plus a list of natural remedies to use when the fever really is too high.

# ACID REFLUX (GERD)

**Quick Fix**

∞ **Apple cider vinegar,** a teaspoonful in a little water or juice, before each meal, or

∞ **Betaine hydrochloride** (hydrochloric acid), a capsule before each meal. Sound scary? It's not. The capsule protects your throat while you swallow it, and hydrochloric acid is what your stomach normally secretes to help you digest your food.

These substances both work on the same principle: the body *needs* hydrochloric acid in the stomach to digest protein and absorb minerals; we produce less and less as we get older; and acid reflux is caused by *lack* of enough acid to trigger the ring of muscles at the top of the stomach and close it off from the esophagus.

This is the opposite principle from the one that conventional medicine uses (the belief that acid reflux is caused by *too much* stomach acid). The proof of the pudding, so to speak, is in the results.

My clients who have tried apple cider vinegar or betaine hydrochloride have reported immediate results and have not needed to repeat it at every meal.

**Lifestyle Support**

Support your digestive system by eating simpler meals and more raw foods, which contain enzymes that can help form your own digestive enzymes. If you just can't incorporate more raw foods, use digestive enzymes made from raw plant enzymes such as ReNew Life's DigestMore.

Be sure to follow the healthy eating guidelines in Part One. Eat sitting down. Take a few deep breaths to center yourself before you eat. Offer thanks if you are so inclined. Eat peacefully and chew slowly. Don't eat right before going to sleep, as you are likely to gain weight as well as having your stomach contents flow back up on you (acid reflux).

Babies with reflux should first be taken off cow's milk, as this may be enough to end the reflux without medication.

# ACNE

## Quick Fix

**A clay mask** such as Queen Helene Mint Julep Mask or Mud Mask. Clay dries up pimples by drawing them out from under the skin and providing minerals to the skin which help it heal. Dab it on problem spots or apply to the whole face. It will dry and get flaky after about 20 minutes, then you just wash it off with warm water, leaving your skin feeling soft and silky. Do problem areas daily, your whole face weekly.

## Ongoing Care

Your skin is trying to tell you something. A healthy body will not have acne. Address one or more of these:

- ∾ Hormonal imbalance, especially in a teenager or in a woman if acne gets worse before/during the period. Increase **essential fatty acids** with a supplement such as Nordic Naturals Ultimate Omega. (A young man who was fed soy formula as a baby may need natural hormone balancing supplements only available to a professional).
- ∾ Eliminate cow's milk products (see page 13).
- ∾ You may need to do an **internal cleansing**. The body eliminates toxins through the skin, especially when the colon and liver are backed up. Talk to the staff at your local health food store about herbs for cleansing the colon and liver, and while you're at it, the blood and lymph (which help carry away the toxins).
- ∾ Replenish your friendly bacteria with a good **probiotic** such as Klaire Ther-Biotic, Jarro-Dophilus or MegaFood's MegaFlora.
- ∾ Take supplements for a healthy skin. The simplest way is to get a combination of vitamins, minerals, and herbs for the skin such as MegaFoods' Skin, Nails and Hair Formula.
- ∾ If your skin tends to get pimples and other infections which are slow to heal, use the cell salt **Silicea** (see page 178). If it tends to form pimples with thick yellowish pus which take a long time to drain, use **Calc. sulph**. (see page 177). For a big pimple, you can actually use the tooth infection series on page 134.

## ALLERGIES/HAYFEVER

**Quick Fix**

Get a **combination homeopathic remedy** for the substance you are allergic to. My favorite products are the **bioAllers series from NatraBio.** They cover not only pollen allergies but also food and pet hair allergies. They are available in any health food store and many drug stores, and they include:

- Pet Allergy, and Animal Hair/Dander (basically the same formula—both cover cat, dog, horse and wool allergies, but the former includes birds while the latter includes cows)
- Dairy Allergies and Grain and Wheat Allergies
- Pollen/Hayfever, Grass Pollen, Tree Pollen, and Outdoor Allergy
- Indoor Allergy, and Mold, Yeast & Dust

Other excellent brands include Pollinosan, Sabadil, and Hyland's Hayfever. Ask your local health food store staff for the best brand for your area, since this will vary depending on your climate and your local pollen-producing vegetation.

**Ongoing Care**

- **Quercetin,** a plant-based flavonoid, can shift your allergic tendencies and reduce your symptoms (250 to 500 mg a day).
- **Vitamin C** (several thousand units a day) and 800 IU a day of **Vitamin E** may also be helpful.
- The herb **butterbur** may work for allergies (take one capsule three times a day, with each capsule containing 8 mg of the isolated active ingredient petasin).

A specific homeopathic remedy that matches your symptoms is likely to give more lasting relief than one of the combination remedies above. For example:

- **Arsenicum** or **Allium cepa:** "nose running like a faucet" with watery discharge; lots of sneezing; "red mustache" under your nose because it's irritated by the discharge.

∾ **Nux vomica:** the nose feels stuffed up, so you can't breathe through it, but you can't blow anything out either, because the tissues inside your nose are swollen up. You also tend to be itchy: itchy eyes, itchy nose, even itchy ears, so you might bore your fingers into your ears.

∾ **Pulsatilla:** your symptoms (stuffed up or runny? clear or white or yellow mucus?) are constantly changing.

∾ **Phosphorus:** tendency to sneeze from fumes and fragrances.

∾ **Sabadilla** for a "salvo of sneezes," one after the other, you just can't stop sneezing.

## Preventing Recurrence

The herb **nettles** can both treat and prevent allergies; for best results, get the freeze-dried form from Oregon's Wild Harvest or Eclectic Institute.

Better yet, just a single dose of **Psorinum** ("sore-EYE-num"), a homeopathic medicine, can work to prevent allergies for an entire season. You have to take it in advance, though. Get a 30c strength (you'll probably have to order it online, as it's an unusual remedy) and take a single dose of a few pellets, about 10 days to two weeks before the start of allergy season.

Keep your tube of Psorinum on hand and mark your calendar so you remember to take it in time. If you get hayfever twice a year, in spring and late summer/early fall, you will need to take Psorinum before each of your hayfever seasons.

Many of my clients, even those who suffer terribly during hayfever season, have reported that they have not even sneezed once during the whole season based on this simple remedy.

If you forget, though, and you start getting symptoms, it's probably too late for Psorinum. Try it anyway and it may take the edge off your symptoms, but you will probably also need one of the other herbs and/or remedies mentioned here.

If Psorinum does not work for you, a holistic health care practitioner should be able to turn around your allergic tendencies, and you will probably notice that other health problems improve at the same time. Look for a functional medicine doctor, a naturopath, or a professional homeopath (pages 237–240).

## ANXIETY

**Quick Fix**

∽ **A GABA formula** like Natural Factors PharmaGABA.

∽ **Rescue Remedy** (page 87).

∽ Homeopathic blends Calms Forte, Sedalia, or Liddell Anxiety Oral Spray.

∽ Breathe as slowly and deeply as you can. Deep breathing helps to calm your system, just as anxiety makes your chest tight and your breathing shallow. Inhaling the fragrance of rose oil makes it luscious!

**Ongoing Care**

∽ The herbs passionflower, wild oats, hops, and chamomile are traditional **calming herbs** contained in the Calms Forte formula recommended above, in mildly potentized (homeopathically energized) doses for best results. They can also be taken in an herbal blend. If you prefer a hot cup of herbal tea, chamomile is a good choice, especially if you have trouble sleeping when you are anxious.

∽ Kava kava, valerian and St. John's wort are additional herbs traditionally used for calming. (Some people seem to be sensitive to valerian and report a sort of reverse effect from it: they don't sleep as well and they wake up with a feeling of mental dullness, almost like a hangover.)

∽ **Magnesium** has a calming effect for many people, and an easy way to take it is in powder form: Natural Calm, which can be stirred into water to make a lemon-flavored drink.

∽ The **B vitamins** are also really important for your mental health. Take a multivitamin that contains a lot of B vitamins (50 to 75 mg of each) and consider taking extra inositol and B3. The B3 (niacin) should be in the form of niacinamide so that it does not cause flushing and a pins-and-needles sensation.

The single homeopathic medicine that matches you best will give you greater relief than the more generic combination remedies Calms Forte and Sedalia. See pages 204 to 208 for more information on how to take these medicines. For example:

**Aconite:** for people with sudden panic attacks, which might include the feeling that they are about to die. It's also used for physical problems that come on suddenly, typically around midnight, perhaps with heart palpitations and/or a high fever. Aconite is most commonly used when fear of dying accompanies an acute physical complaint (and it can often resolve both the physical and emotional symptoms). It is sometimes used when the problem is primarily emotional, such as panic attacks with heart palpitations.

**Arsenicum:** for people with many fears related to survival—fear of illness, of dying, of not having enough money, of losing their job, of becoming homeless. These fears may seem groundless to anyone else but may seem overwhelming to people who need Arsenicum. These people also tend to be neat freaks and control freaks. They may also be parents hovering over their children and fretting over every possible germ exposure.

**Argentum nitricum:** for people with specific fears (flying, going over bridges) where the person has a vivid imagination for what might go wrong ("What if *this* happens? What if *that* happens?"). If the person has the typical physical symptoms of Argentum nitricum, it is especially likely to work. These include rumbling intestinal gas and explosive diarrhea. Sometimes fear of not finding a bathroom is the biggest fear!

**Gelsemium:** most often used for fear of the dentist, fear of going to the doctor, fear of medical tests, fear of exams, and even for pets who have a fear of the vet. (How do they know they're going to the vet?) People who need Gelsemium express their anxiety with a numb, brain-dead, "deer in the headlights" kind of quality, and they may feel totally drained of energy with droopy eyelids as if they are about to fall asleep. They may get diarrhea because their anal sphincter is also too relaxed.

**Lycopodium:** most often used for fear of public speaking, although Gelsemium will work better if the physical symptoms match better. People who need Lycopodium tend to have digestive symptoms, especially intestinal gas. The basic feeling with Lycopodium is "I'm not big enough for the job. I'm not qualified for what I've been asked to do."

I've used it for clients who have been promoted, with full confidence from their manager, but who feel like imposters in their new position.

## Lifestyle Support

These suggestions are meant to help with occasional or mild anxiety. If anxiety is a major ongoing problem for you, homeopathy is likely to help, but it's beyond the scope of self-care. A professional homeopath can find the best match for you from among hundreds of medicines, many of which are not available over-the-counter.

If you would like to know more about how professional homeopathic care can help heal your emotional symptoms, consult Robert Ullman and Judyth Reichenberg-Ullman's *Prozac-Free*. It's not a self-help book, however its vivid case stories will give you a sense of what professional treatment can do.

If you have ongoing major anxiety you'll need nutritional support too, which you can learn about from Dr. Mark Hyman's excellent book, *The UltraMind Solution: Fix Your Broken Brain by Healing Your Body First—The Simple Way to Defeat Depression, Overcome Anxiety, and Sharpen Your Mind*.

# ARTHRITIS

## Quick Fix

**Topricin** or **Traumeel** are excellent formulas which can relieve the pain of arthritis. Both are available as creams to apply topically, and Traumeel is also available as tablets to take internally. Both cover a wide range of traumas and injuries.

The ingredients in **Castro's Joint Cream** are specifically targeted to joint symptoms and may provide better relief for some people.

## Ongoing Care

Nutritional supplements are also essential. While they typically cannot provide the instant relief that homeopathic medicines sometimes can, they quietly work to give your joints the nutrients needed for healing. Here are some of the best:

- **Curcumin** and **bromelain** are excellent anti-inflammatory supplements. You can get them combined in a Natural Factors product.
- **Glucosamine** helps repair your joints (1500 mg a day) while **chondroitin** reduces pain and increases your range of motion (1200 mg a day). You can easily find supplements that combine the two.
- **Omega-3 essential fatty acids** will also reduce inflammation. Nordic Naturals is an excellent brand: try their Ultimate Omega.
- **SAMe**, well known as a natural antidepressant, also helps with the pain of arthritis (1200 mg a day), as does the sulfur compound **MSM** (2250 mg a day).
- **Anti-oxidants** found in richly-colored fruits and vegetables will help, as recommended in Part One.

The specific homeopathic medicine that matches your particular symptoms may provide more lasting relief than the creams listed above:

- **Rhus tox.** is the most common homeopathic medicine for arthritis because it matches the typical "rusty gate" symptoms: you feel stiff when you first wake up or first try to get up from a chair, you need to limber up, then you can move just fine—except if you keep moving too long, your joints are painful again. People who need Rhus tox. tend to feel better from warmth (a hot bath or heating pad) and worse from damp.

∞ **Ruta grav.** works for similar symptoms, so if Rhus tox. does not work for you, try Ruta grav. instead.

∞ **Bryonia** works for the opposite symptoms: feeling worse from the slightest movement and the tendency to "guard" or "splint" a joint to prevent the motion which causes pain.

There are many other herbs and supplements that have been found helpful for arthritis, too many to list here but easily available at your local health food store.

### Lifestyle Support

Arthritis is the result of a general inflammatory condition in your body from our terrible American diet and other lifestyle factors.

Dr. Mark Hyman's *Ultra Inflammation: How to Cool the Fire Inside That's Making You Fat and Diseased* will explain the causes of arthritis and how to truly cure it with changes in your diet and lifestyle. The book will help you lose weight, have more energy, and gain such a positive outlook that the disappearance of your arthritis symptoms may seem like just a side benefit.

# ATHLETE'S FOOT

## Quick Fix

Thuja is a natural antifungal medicine which can be taken internally or applied externally. It's better to apply it topically unless you need it systemically. If you have a systemic fungal infection such as candida, or if your body has a general tendency to produce warts, polyps, and other growths, then it would make sense to take it internally (see instructions on pages 204–208).

Otherwise, dissolve a couple of pellets of the 30c potency in a small amount of water (for example, fill a clean plastic deli container) and soak your feet for 10 minutes twice a day. This technique will also work for fungus under the nails.

## Ongoing Care

Herbal options include tea tree oil and garlic. Unfortunately these options are smelly, and they tend to take longer than Thuja. But if Thuja does not work for you, try this:

Use a cream with 10% **tea tree oil**. Or if you have concentrated 100% tea tree oil, make your own 10% solution in a mild oil such as olive oil. (Tea tree oil straight up is likely to be too strong for your skin and may cause a burning sensation.)

**Garlic** is a powerful antifungal and could be minced fine then added to a cream, or to olive oil, and rubbed on the feet, leading to the question, which is worse — fungal feet or feet that smell like garlic?

## Preventing Recurrence

Fungal infections like to grow where it is warm, dark, and damp. So you want to keep your feet dry: apply a powder to your feet to absorb the sweat, and change socks when they are sweaty. Go barefoot at home and try to give your feet some time in the sunlight, which has natural fungal-repelling properties. (Try using your athlete's foot as an excuse for medical leave to spend time at the beach!)

## BACK PAIN

**Quick Fix**

- Use **Rescue Remedy** spray on the injured spot, and also spray it in your mouth.
- **Liddell's BPS** ("back pain + sciatica") provides a blend of homeopathic medicines in a fast-acting oral spray.
- You can also use the same creams and homeopathic medicines recommended for **Arthritis**. The nutritional supplements are different, though, if your back pain is from injury rather than arthritis.

**Ongoing Care**

Nutritional supplements can help repair the damage to your back. This protocol will only work for the first few days after you injure your back. Here's what you can do for an acute injury (one that just happened):

- **Omega-3 fatty acids** such as Nordic Naturals Ultimate Omega: take double the amount because that will help reduce inflammation.
- **Digestive enzymes:** if you're not already taking them, get a good digestive enzyme with papain such as ReNew Life's DigestMore. Take the recommended amount four times a day, away from meals. That means at least 30 minutes before eating and at least two hours after eating a meal. Otherwise the digestive enzyme will get used up helping you digest your food, whereas you want them to help reduce inflammation around your back injury.

If back pain becomes a chronic problem, you really need to see a chiropractor. However, you can alleviate the pain with supplements like these:

- A **curcumin** supplement to reduce inflammation, such as Terry Naturally Curamin, which includes curcumin and other natural pain relievers.
- Rainbow Light Pain-Eze with traditional **pain-relieving herbs** like California poppy, peony, and meadowsweet.

A homeopathic medicine can provide lasting pain relief (although it cannot provide permanent relief if the problem is primarily structural, requiring a chiropractor). **Rhus tox.** and **Bryonia**, described in the Arthritis section, are among the most common remedies for back pain. Or try one of these, whichever matches best, and see pages 204–208 for instructions:

- **Nux vomica:** a great remedy for lower back pain, especially in the typical Nux type person (ambitious, competitive, driven, with a tendency to use stimulants like cigarettes, coffee, spicy foods, or drugs to keep going). One typical symptom: they can't roll over in bed, they have to sit up instead, due to their back pain.

- **Sepia:** when the back pain is hormonal, during a woman's menstrual cycle. See **Hormone Balancing** for more about this remedy.

- **Aesculus:** for pain in the sacro-iliac joint (a "pain in the butt" several inches on either side of the spine). The person has a hard time getting out of a chair because the area is so stiff.

- **Helodrilus** is such an unusual homeopathic medicine, it's not in retail stores but it's worth ordering. It's a great remedy for back pain and it has a special ability to help repair slipped and herniated disks. No promises (depends on how badly damaged your disks are) but worth a try, and in my experience it sometimes helps.

For more specialized information on back pain, see *Homeopathy for Musculoskeletal Problems* by Dr. Asa Hershoff.

### Preventing Recurrence

If you tend to injure your back a lot, you may need to strengthen the muscles around it, for example with weight training (low weight, high reps). It's always wise to get a personal trainer to create a program for you if you're injured.

Or you may need to learn how to hold yourself with better posture and use better ergonomics at work. A Feldenkrais or Alexander practitioner may be able to help you by providing greater awareness of your posture and teaching more efficient movements (**www.Feldenkrais .com**, **www.AlexanderTech.com**).

A chiropractor may be able to adjust something in your skeletal structure to help prevent future injuries. The chiropractors I work with recommend finding a chiropractor who uses a non-force technique (activator method), and ideally someone who does Sacro-Occipital Technique with applied kinesiology, to get the best results. I often refer my clients to my colleagues, even if my clients have been going to other chiropractors for years without lasting results. They often get better quickly with this combination of techniques. For a chiropractor near you using the non-force technique, see **www.Activator.com**, and for those using the Sacro-Occipital Technique, see **www.SORSI.com**.

I know people who have overcome chronic, untreatable back pain with the techniques described in *Healing Back Pain: The Mind-Body Connection* by John E. Sarno, MD, based on the concept that back pain is due to tension from repressed emotions. Apparently increased awareness of the underlying psychosomatic reason for back pain has been enough to relieve it successfully in thousands of people without the need for drugs or surgery.

I know many others who have had success with the Egoscue Method. The exercises are so simple (they often involve just lying down in a specific position supported by blocks or props) it's hard to believe how well they work.

When I was running a lot of marathons, the Egoscue method spread like wildfire in my running community because it was so effective. Learn more from the book, *Pain-Free Living* by Pete Egoscue, or check YouTube for demonstration videos. For best results get your own customized program from an Egoscue trainer, either by visiting a local Egoscue center or by uploading photos of your posture to the website, **www.Egoscue.com**.

# BEDWETTING

## Quick Fix

**Bedwetting Tabs** by Hylands are a generic formula, likely to help in many cases.

## Ongoing Care

- **Pulsatilla** for bedwetting in children *if* they have the typical Pulsatilla personality (cuddly and affectionate, clingy to mom, mostly sweet tempered but sometimes whiny and manipulative) and *if* they seem to be acting babyish in general—for example if a new baby is getting all the attention—or *if* they seem to feel abandoned, especially by mom. Pulsatilla is the most common remedy for bedwetting in my experience, but it's not likely to work if these symptoms don't match. If they do, Pulsatilla is likely to resolve your child's whole emotional/behavioral complex and support more age-appropriate behavior.

  See pages 204–208 for instructions. For other homeopathic medicines for bedwetting that might be a better fit, see Dana Ullman's *Homeopathic Medicines for Children and Infants*.

- **Equisetum** as a homeopathic medicine, for example in the formula **Be-Dry** by Native Remedies.

- **Equisetum** (horsetail) as an *herbal tincture* strengthens the muscles of the bladder and helps improve control. Give a dropperful twice a day in water or juice. It can be used in addition to any homeopathic medicine for bedwetting.

**Chiropractic adjustments:** If these natural medicines don't work, chiropractic adjustments may help with bladder problems in small children, especially if the child has had an injury to the lower back (where the nerves come out that go to the bowel and bladder). You might think your child never had an injury there, but . . . did she ever fall off the changing table, for example? It happens. It doesn't mean you're a bad mother.

Or the pubic bones may have gotten pushed up when your child landed on her crotch (say on a fence, gymnastics equipment, or the crossbar of a bike). My colleagues at Lydian Chiropractic have cured many a case of bedwetting that started with an injury.

Maybe you're not aware of a particular injury (kids fall all the time, and most of the time they're fine). But think of this approach if a child suddenly loses potty training. If your child has been dry for a year and suddenly is back in diapers again, there must be a reason.

Find a non-force chiropractor who uses applied kinesiology and has experience working with kids. Applied kinesiology will help the chiropractor sleuth out what happened to your child, even if you don't know the cause. Non-force chiropractic is safe for kids because it's so gentle, they won't even feel the chiropractor touching them.

## BLEEDING AND BRUISING

### Quick Fix for Bleeding

෴ **Phosphorus** as a homeopathic medicine has often stopped bleeding in its tracks, in my experience with my clients. It can stop a nosebleed, or heavy menstrual bleeding, or bleeding from a tooth extraction, or a cut that just won't stop bleeding. It's especially likely to work for bright red bleeding.

෴ **Hamamelis** is more likely to work if the bleeding is darker colored and slower moving—in other words, from a vein.

### Quick Fix for Bruises

෴ **Arnica** or **Traumeel** taken internally (see pages 204–208).

෴ **Arnica, Traumeel,** or **Topricin** ointment applied externally.

You can use both internal and topical treatments at the same time for faster results.

### Preventing Recurrence

If you tend to bleed or bruise easily, you may need to strengthen the walls of your blood vessels with these supplements:

෴ **Calc. fluor. 6x,** a tissue salt (see p. 174) for strengthening elastic tissues like blood vessel walls.

෴ **Rutin,** part of the vitamin C complex. You can buy it separately, but better yet, look for Vitamin C with bioflavonoids, then read the fine print on the label. The ones that *specify* the rutin content will contain more than ones that simply list bioflavonoids in general. Or you can eat foods high in rutin such as

  ○ the white on the inside of citrus fruit peel

  ○ black, green, or rooibos tea

  ○ buckwheat or kasha (a fabulous source of plant-based protein which would be a great addition to your meals anyway. You probably already know the smoky flavor from buckwheat pancakes.)

## BLISTERS

**Quick Fix**

For blisters, while the conventional wisdom is to pop the blister with a sterilized needle, others feel that a blister is nature's most perfect way to protect the area with a little padding and sterile fluid. During a marathon or long run, you should only pop a blister that is big, juicy and tight—in other words, one that is about to pop anyway. Popping it under controlled circumstances (with a sterile lancet or a needle soaked in rubbing alcohol) allows you to clean the area with alcohol, then dress it as described below.

**Cantharis** is a good remedy to take internally for blistered skin (instructions for homeopathics on pages 204–208).

**Ongoing Care**

**Calendula cream** or **Seven Cream** will help heal any blistered area.

**Preventing Recurrence**

If you tend to blister easily, you can use a chafing cream like **Badger Balm**. You can also protect a hot spot (where a blister is likely to form) with moleskin or **Spenco Second Skin**, a thin layer of gel-like substance. Runners can hold it on with paper tape (for short races or runs) or silk tape (which lasts better for long races but can bunch up a bit more in your running shoes). Painting the surrounding skin with tincture of benzoin before taping helps hold the whole thing in place while you're running.

For blisters between the toes (I'm thinking of runners and other athletes here), rub Badger Balm between the toes, then surround each toe with tufts of lambs wool. If you get blisters between your toes because your feet sweat there, try **Silicea 6x** (the cell salt, page 178) or **Silica 30c** (the homeopathic remedy). **Silicea 6x** is fine for daily use longterm. **Silica 30c** is stronger, best used occasionally for prevention right before a race, a long run or a tennis game on a hot day.

# BREASTFEEDING

## Quick Fix

**For a blocked milk duct:** the homeopathic medicine **Silica,** and hold the baby in a "football hold" while breastfeeding.

## For cracked or sore nipples:

∾ **Natural Nipple Butter** (contains Calendula and natural oils).

∾ any **comfrey ointment.**

∾ The homeopathic medicine **Graphites,** easily available in stores, or **Castor equi** (may work better but will probably need to be special-ordered). Taken internally, they will work from the inside out.

**For thrush:** Are you and your baby passing thrush back and forth? It may show up as little white patches inside your baby's mouth, and your nipples may be painful, itchy, or flaky. The homeopathic medicine **Borax** can help both of you. It's safe for babies (see page 209).

## Lifestyle Support

Take good care of your breasts. You can start before your baby is even born to get your nipples in good shape. Massaging with **comfrey ointment** is a great habit to get into, before the birth.

Hot compresses feel wonderful and can help loosen things up, especially if you tend to get blocked milk ducts. Apply a hot washcloth to the area for a few minutes before each feeding.

Thrush is a form of candida, which thrives in warm, dark, moist areas. There's no getting around the fact that your baby's mouth is an ideal environment, but you can prevent thrush from growing on your breasts by keeping them dry.

Here are a couple of informative books:

∾ *Wise Woman Herbal for the Childbearing Year* by Susan Weed.

∾ *Homeopathic Medicines for Pregnancy, Birth, and Baby's First Year* by Miranda Castro.

# BURNS AND SUNBURN

## Quick Fix

∽ **Calendula spray** is easily available in health food stores. The spray form allows this skin-healing plant to be applied without touching the burned area. Calendula can help prevent pain, infection and scarring.

∽ **Aloe vera gel** will soothe the pain and help heal a burn or sunburn if the person doesn't mind the area being touched. Keeping aloe vera gel in the refrigerator will give it an extra cooling effect. When the burn is extremely painful, you can get aloe vera mixed with a conventional anesthetic such as lidocaine (for example **Solarcaine**).

The best-matching homeopathic medicine can be taken internally at the same time (see pages 204-208 for directions):

∽ **Calendula** is also used internally so that it can work systemically for any skin condition covering a large area. Use for first-degree burns.

∽ **Cantharis** is better when there is blistering from burns or sunburn, and **Causticum** for chemical burns.

## Ongoing Care

**Sol** is a homeopathic medicine which can sometimes reverse sun damage. It's an unusual remedy and will need to be ordered online, for example from **www.Homeopathic.com**. Ask for **Sol California** in a mild 6c potency and take a few pellets daily until the sun damage is gone (or stop after a month if nothing has changed). I have seen it reverse sun-damaged skin, for example small dark keloids on the face of an African-American woman.

## Preventing Recurrence

Antioxidants such as **vitamins C and E** plus the carotenoid **lycopene** (found in tomato sauce) can protect against sunburns.

# CANCER TREATMENT, SIDE EFFECTS OF

## Quick Fix

**For nausea caused by chemotherapy:**

Nux vomica, easily available in stores. If it does not work, try a more unusual one that you will need to get online: **Cadmium sulph.** Either way, take a preventive dose immediately before each treatment and afterwards as needed. (Follow the directions on page 211.)

## For the side effects of radiation therapy:

Calendula can be used for radiation burns. This treatment is so effective that many cancer centers are now recommending homeopathic Calendula ointment to patients undergoing radiation.

Calendula can also be made into a mouthwash for people who develop sores in their mouth and throat during head-neck radiation. These sores are a serious problem: they are so painful that they can interfere with swallowing and thereby contribute to the weight loss and wasting associated with cancer. See page 208 for how to make a solution with a homeopathic medicine. Calendula in water can be swished like mouthwash, then safely swallowed to treat sores in the esophagus.

The homeopathic medicines **X-ray** and **Radium bromatum** are worth special ordering. They protect against other side effects of both chemotherapy and radiation, including severe fatigue and weakness. They also protect against radiation burns when taken internally.

## Ongoing Care

*Embrace, Release, Heal* by Leigh Forston is an excellent introduction to alternative treatments for cancer. She sought out an alternative treatment for herself, when her cancer returned for a third time and her doctors told her there was nothing more they could do.

After healing herself, she went on to interview several dozen other people who had used natural methods to heal their cancer. Most were either doing conventional treatment simultaneously but were told they had only a small chance of survival, or they were told that their cancer could not be treated by conventional medicine. (In other words, they were not refusing conventional treatment in favor of alternative treatment.)

Forston was surprised at how easy it was to find people who had survived cancer through alternative treatments, and also surprised that her oncologist was not allowed to tell other patients about Forston's recovery. The methods described in the book cover the full gamut from raw foods to internal cleansing to prayer circles to intravenous therapy at a clinic in Mexico.

In addition to the inspiring personal stories of many cancer survivors, the book includes interviews with the healers whose methods were used, plus practical information on how to schedule treatment with them.

Another uplifting book about overcoming cancer with a natural approach is *Anti-Cancer: A New Way of Life* by Dr. David Servan-Schreiber. A physician who co-founded Doctors Without Borders and the Center for Integrative Medicine at the University of Pittsburgh Medical Center, Dr. Servan-Schreiber conducted an intensive study of the anti-cancer effects of foods, supplements, and lifestyle factors that would reduce the risk of cancer. He was highly motivated—his own brain tumor had returned and he was able to keep his "terminal" cancer at bay for 15 years with the methods in this book. Servan-Schreiber explains how cancer works—that's empowering in itself—then goes on to suggest many ways to prevent or fend off cancer.

# CANKER SORES

## Quick Fix

∾ **Calendula** is a bit of a cure-all for canker sores (little sores inside the mouth, whether they represent little spots of infection, or little cuts from braces or dentures). Calendula can stop infection and heal the skin anywhere that it is cut. You can put a few drops of herbal Calendula tincture, or a few pellets of homeopathic Calendula, into a little water. Stir well, swish like mouthwash, and swallow.

∾ **Aloe vera** can also be healing and soothing. **George's Always Active Aloe Vera** is an excellent brand. It looks and tastes like water but it has strong medicinal properties.

## Ongoing Care

If you keep getting canker sores, the best matching homeopathic medicine is likely to help heal them, prevent them, and possibly help other things in your body at the same time. For example:

∾ **Mercurius** is not only a great medicine for canker sores, it covers a lot of problems in the mouth: bleeding or infected gums, bad breath, excessive salivation, and a metallic taste in your mouth. Here's a quick way to tell if you need it: look in the mirror, stick out your tongue, and hold it sideways. If it's scalloped along the edge, indented by your teeth, you are likely to need this medicine. You are especially likely to need it after mercury exposure, for example if you just had an old filling replaced.

∾ **Arsenicum:** When Arsenicum is needed anywhere in the body, there is likely to be a burning sensation. It's especially likely to help canker sores if the person is fretting over them like a typical Arsenicum personality: see page 184.

∾ **Nat. mur.,** a homeopathic preparation of salt, is used (not surprisingly) when the lips and mouth are very dry and the person craves salt. It can also help even if none of these physical conditions are present but the person has the psychological profile of Nat. mur. (silent grief, protecting the wounded heart, reserved, holding potential close relationships at arms' length, working hard and taking life seriously, with easily hurt feelings).

∾ **Borax** is used for thrush, the little white patches in the mouth that represent fungal infections, often passed back and forth between baby and nursing mother.

No matter which of these medicines you use, you can also use your Calendula or aloe mouthwash to heal your current sores, and they may also act as a preventive if used regularly.

## Preventing Recurrence

If you get canker sores frequently, you may be low in **B vitamins, iron,** or **zinc**. If you're not taking a good multivitamin, start with that, then add extra nutrients if necessary.

Canker sores can also be caused by food allergies, especially a gluten sensitivity.

# COLDS AND NASAL CONGESTION

## Quick Fix

Stop a cold when it first starts, in the watery-drippy phase, with Arsenicum or Allium cepa. **Arsenicum** is the most common medicine in my practice for the "nose running like a faucet" stage of colds, so I would try it first.

**Allium cepa** is a good backup especially if you have an itchy nose or red raw skin under the nose, a "red mustache."

You might be able to nip your cold in the bud with **Ferrum phos.** (page 170).

Or use **Xlear** nasal spray. Can't pronounce it? Doesn't matter. It's a saline rinse with the added benefit of xylitol, a safe natural birch bark extract which stops the growth of bacteria in your nasal passages. Works for sinus congestion too, as does **Sinusin**, the homeopathic blend by BHI Heel (for nasal and sinus congestion).

Another option for clearing out congestion: rinse with a **neti pot**, which looks like a little Aladdin's lamp and is used to clear out the nasal passages. Just be sure to use distilled water and sterilize the pot between uses (for example by running it through the dishwasher). Many of my clients find their neti pot easy and effective to use, but I would try Xlear or Sinusin first. If they work for you, they're much simpler than a neti pot.

## Ongoing Care

Meanwhile, get your supplements and herbs going:

- ✎ **Zinc lozenges,** ideally blended with the mineral selenium which has been called "birth control for viruses" like the cold virus.
- ✎ **Extra vitamin C,** up to 1000 mg per hour.
- ✎ **Immune herbs** like andrographis, echinacea, goldenseal, astragalus (your health food store can recommend a good combination).
- ✎ **The amino acid lysine,** well known for killing the herpes virus, also works against the cold virus.
- ✎ **A good probiotic,** with *billions* (not millions) of organisms per capsule.

The middle phase of a cold with medium thick, rattly mucus has several possible homeopathic medicines. Try **Hepar sulph.**, especially if the person is sensitive to cold and drafts and/or is irritable and wants to be left alone. Try **Pulsatilla** for a child who fits the overall personality type (mild tempered, affectionate, clingy to mom, a little whiny, with moods quickly changing from tears to smiles).

The last phase, with thick sticky mucus ("boogers") responds well to **Kali bic.** (rhymes with Bic pens, as in "If it sticks, use Kali bic."). This particular homeopathic medicine is so effective against so many boogery conditions (thick mucus in the ears, nose, throat, lungs, around the larynx) that it should be part of everyone's home remedy kit.

## Preventing Recurrence

Try to remember how you felt the day before you got the cold, so you can "nip it in the bud" next time with **Ferrum phos.** (page 170) before it even has a chance to settle in.

During a season when you tend to get sick a lot, it's wise to help out your immune system by minimizing things that weaken it (sugar, stress) and increasing things that strengthen it (essential fatty acids, herbs like echinacea, bilberry, andrographis). You don't have to pronounce these herbs. Any health food store will have a good immune-strengthening "wellness formula."

I like **Zand's Insure Herbal** — it was the big favorite in my store. It has echinacea and goldenseal, the traditional "stars" of immune-boosting herbs, with a "supporting cast" of a dozen other herbs. Remember that if you take a stimulating herb year round, it will lose its "oomph" because your body will get used to it. Save it for when you really need it — when you get run down, when someone close to you is sick, or when you're actually sick.

# CONSTIPATION

## Quick Fix

An herbal laxative containing **senna** or **cascara sagrada** can work quickly (as in, stay near a bathroom) but should only be used very occasionally. These herbs stimulate the muscles of the colon and send them into spasm, which relieves the situation temporarily. But over-stimulation can actually weaken the muscles of the colon, making the problem worse in the long run.

## Ongoing Care

This depends on the reason for constipation. Are you drinking enough water and eating enough fiber-containing fruits and vegetables? If not, that's a good place to start.

An easy way to add fiber is with **psyllium powder** (which you may already be familiar with as Metamucil, but you can get it in bulk in your health food store without the sugar or aspartame). Stir a teaspoon into a glass of water and drink it fast before it sets up into a gel, then follow it with another full glass of water, or else it could actually make things more sluggish. It is a gentle cleansing fiber that will tend to push everything right on through and come out the other end as huge, puffy, floating coils of stuff.

Psyllium by itself is often not enough, though. Usually it works best in tandem with colon cleansing herbs. Your local health food store will have a wide selection.

For some people, especially children, eliminating cow's milk is essential. In one study, eliminating cow's milk was enough to get small kids pooping regularly.

Your friendly bacteria are also important. Did you know that in terms of the number of cells, your body is mostly bacteria? Like it or not, it's true, and you might as well make sure you've got the friendly ones in there. You do that by taking a good **probiotic** such as Klaire Ther-Biotic Complete, Jarro-Dophilus or MegaFood's MegaFlora. You also want to create a friendly environment for your little friends, or else they will be driven out by the unfriendly bacteria, the ones that contribute to disease, and you definitely don't want that. There are so many factors in our modern life that tend to favor the unfriendly bacteria: sugar, alcohol, sodas, meat, processed foods, lack of fiber, antibiotics, anything that affects the acid-alkaline balance, and even if you're a purist and have perfect diet, your internal environment is still affected by stress. The healthy lifestyle suggestions in Part One of this book will help, in particular:

- ∾ Plenty of **good oils and fats** such as coconut oil, olive oil and organic butter or ghee, both used in cooking and added to each meal.
- ∾ **Vita-Mix smoothies** with both fruits and vegetables, because you will get their nutritional benefits with the fiber included, which can help prevent constipation.
- ∾ **Raw vegetable juices** are good in a different way if you are really backed up, because the juices will absorb readily (giving you concentrated nutrition) and there will be no extra fiber to add uncomfortably to the traffic jam in your colon.
- ∾ **Fermented foods** such as kefir, fresh sauerkraut, miso.

Maybe your constipation problem is partly a biomechanical problem. The human body was not made to poop sitting upright on a toilet. Humans have traditionally squatted, and up until recently you would find squat toilets (nicely tiled) even in advanced civilizations like Europe and Japan. As American toilets have taken over, not to mention American food, constipation has followed in their wake, followed by phones in hotel bathrooms for constipated businessmen.

So here's what you do. If you can, put your feet on your toilet seat and hug your knees to your chest. Beginner's version: keep a low stool by the toilet so your feet are elevated off the ground. Advanced version: massage your abdomen while you're sitting there waiting for some action.

Visualize your colon. It starts on your right side, down by the crease between your abdomen and your legs, then it travels up towards your ribs, across your belly to the left side, down the left side to the crease by your legs, then it takes a little turn to end up in the middle by your anus, or as your kids probably call it, your poop hole. I'm telling you the story of your colon because it will help to massage it all along the route, and you want to be pushing things in the right direction.

**Aloe vera** can help with constipation in several ways: it can stimulate the contraction of the muscles of the colon, soften the stool, and provide bulk. George's Always Active Aloe Vera is remarkable both for its effectiveness and for the fact that it looks and tastes like water, so it's really easy to get down, or to have your child drink.

Another way to provide bulk is with **glucomannan**, a soluble fiber (konjac fiber) that swells up more than 15 times its original volume when water is added. Konjac fiber is the source of shirataki noodles, which provide bulk and a sense of fullness but no calories. (I know, this sounds too good to be true, but they are great for weight loss.)

A castor oil pack is a great way to loosen things up, and it feels great. It will also give you time to relax and ponder your life, which is something we don't take enough time to do. A rush-rush, stressed out lifestyle might be part of the reason you are constipated. See directions for a castor oil pack on page 79.

Speaking of the rush-rush, stressed out lifestyle, if your constipation is related to stress or your emotional state, then homeopathic medicines are your best bet. Use a combo like BHI Heel's Constipation, or your closest-matching single remedy. For example:

∾ **Nux vomica** matches well if you have a Type A personality and a high powered lifestyle. Typically people needing this remedy work long hours and keep themselves going with stimulants such as coffee, cigarettes, spicy foods, junk foods, and drugs. They may be ambitious, competitive, and irritable. Their constipation is characterized by ineffective cramping—the cramping may be painful, but they are left with a feeling that there's still something in there, which makes them crazy.

∾ **Bryonia** is another medicine for a grouchy, constipated businessperson but in this case the problem is dryness—dry mouth, dry rectum, dry bowel movements—and drinking more water doesn't seem to help.

∾ **Nat. mur.** is also for constipation characterized by dryness, but in this case the emotional state is one of longstanding silent grief, grief about a long-ago loss, grief about which the person says, "I never shed a tear." There is a pattern of holding on here: holding on to memories, holding on to a relationship that ended instead of starting a new one, and even holding on in the colon area.

Sound crazy? Actually, scientists have recently discovered what's called "the brain in the gut"—a whole separate branch of the nervous system in the lining of the intestine which is totally plugged in to your emotions. This intersection of the physical and the emotional is an area especially suited to homeopathy.

If none of these homeopathic medicines for constipation match your symptoms, a professional homeopath can help find one for you that will get you going in more ways than one.

If constipation does not respond to these methods, consider **chiropractic care.** My chiropractor colleagues talk about children who have been on Miralax almost since birth, who just need to have their pelvis stabilized. A few adjustments, and the child is having healthy normal bowel movements. Be sure to look for a non-force chiropractor who works with kids.

My chiropractor colleagues say that sometimes the pelvis needs to be stabilized due to an injury, and that the parents may not be aware of the injury since kids fall so much. It can happen to adults, too, who don't make the connection between a fall and the loss of the ability to control bowel movements. Try to find a non-force chiropractor who uses the activator method and applied kinesiology (not as hard as it sounds, these are common techniques).

As another option for kids, check out the GAPS diet (**www.GAPS diet.com**) and Dr. Natasha Campbell-McBride's *Gut and Psychology Syndrome.* Her recommendations are too extreme for most kids and are not necessary unless your child has severe physical problems or is on the autistic spectrum, but you will pick up a lot of important tips from her approach.

# HOW TO MAKE A CASTOR OIL PACK

Castor oil packs have traditionally been used to soften, loosen and break down anything that is hardened or impacted in the body, including constipation, scar tissue, adhesions, and cysts in the breasts. One hypothesis as to their method of action asserts that castor oil on a molecular level has a crystalline structure similar to that of quartz and is able to concentrate healing energies in the way a crystal would.

The basic concept of a castor oil pack is that you want a thick layer of castor oil-soaked flannel next to your skin and a way to apply heat for 20 minutes or more to help it soak in, plus a plastic bag or saran wrap in between to keep the oil from getting on the towel that goes on top of everything to keep the heat in. (Think of a club sandwich with you on the bottom, then the castor-oil soaked flannel, then the saran wrap, then the hot water bottle, and then the towel on top.)

Doing a castor oil pack feels really wonderful. It's great to have a healing modality which is so powerful and feels so good. It takes a little extra effort in the beginning to get the stuff and learn how to do it. It will probably become second nature and a part of your healing "toolkit" which you come back to again and again.

## Specific Instructions

- Get some castor oil, available in 4 oz., 8 oz and 16 oz. bottles. I would get at least 8 oz. if you're planning to do this regularly.
- Also get some wool flannel. These two things are available in good health food stores or could easily be ordered. Home Health is a brand that makes both of them. The wool flannel has special conductive properties and is sold alongside the castor oil.
- Fold the wool flannel so that it is a little larger than the area you want to cover on your body.
- Put it in a glass or ceramic baking dish and pour castor oil on to saturate it.
- Put it in a 350° oven to heat it. (Don't microwave it.) You want it as hot as you can comfortably stand it but not hot enough to burn

you of course. Put it on your skin with a layer of plastic (e.g. plastic bag, saran wrap) over it.

∾ On top of that, place a hot water bottle filled with the hottest water you can get from the tap (or a heated buckwheat pillow, but please no electric heating pads).

∾ And finally a towel to hold the heat in.

Ideally you lie like this for an hour listening to beautiful and inspiring music. Edgar Cayce, the "sleeping prophet," was a great proponent of castor oil packs. He recommended doing it three days in a row each week. You'll just do whatever is possible for your lifestyle.

In between usages, refrigerate the castor oil and the saturated flannel in the little plastic bag it came in.

To remove the oil at the end, it helps to dissolve a teaspoon or two of baking soda in a little warm water to scrub the area, then use soap to get the rest off.

# COUGHS

**Quick Fix**

**Slippery elm** and **elderberry** are great herbs for coughs. They might take care of coughs quickly—slippery elm by soothing, elderberry by acting as an antibacterial and antiviral.

**Slippery elm** comes in throat lozenge form, for example as Two Trees lozenges, or in tea form, such as Traditional Medicinals' Throat Coat tea.

**Elderberry** is delicious in syrup form which gives it a soothing quality. I like supporting local products, so I recommend Maine Medicinals' Antho Immune formula. Or for kids, my favorite is Apitherapy elderberry syrup in honey (honey also has antimicrobial properties). If you can't find these New England brands, look for a national brand like Sambucol. When you're sick, take elderberry syrup by the spoonful. Kids love the fruity taste.

There are many other natural cough syrups. Han's Honey Loquat Syrup, based on Traditional Chinese Medicine, works best for me. There are several good homeopathic blends, such as Hylands, B&T, and Chestal cough syrups.

**Preventing Recurrence**

If you can find a single homeopathic remedy that hits the nail on the head by matching your symptoms, it can work on the spot and also prevent recurrence better than a blend. There are many possibilities. Here are a few that work well for my clients:

- **Bryonia** for a dry cough that hurts so much, you want to hold your chest still so your ribs don't hurt.
- **Phosphorus** for a dry cough triggered by talking or going out into cold air, or by breathing in fumes or fragrances.
- **Rumex** for a dry cough triggered by tickling in your throat pit as if there's a tiny sliver of paper you just can't cough up.
- **Hepar sulph.** for soft rattly mucus right in the middle of the chest.
- **Kali bic.** for thick, sticky mucus you can't cough up.

## CUTS AND SCRAPES

**Quick Fix**

Any time the skin is broken **Calendula** works as a natural antibiotic and pain reliever, plus it joins the sides of a cut together and prevents scarring. You can find it in lotion or spray form. (Spraying is ideal when the skin can't be touched, as for a burn.) Homeopathic or herbal form, doesn't matter. One of the favorite products in my health food store was Weleda Baby Cream with herbal calendula.

The homeopathic pellets have a couple of advantages over the herbal form. They are inexpensive because just a couple of pellets will make a lot of liquid to apply externally. Also, if you have cuts or burns over a large area or different parts of your body, you can take homeopathic Calendula internally and it will work systemically.

The pellets will probably need to be special-ordered, as health food stores don't usually have them. They are among my top recommendations for your home natural medicine cabinet. Dissolve a couple in a little water to apply externally, and take a sip first so that the Calendula can work internally at the same time. You can also wet the gauze of a bandage or dressing in this Calendula water for quick healing.

**Ongoing Care**

If your skin tends to need a long time to heal, take the cell salt **Silicea** 6x (page 178).

**Seven Cream** is even better than Calendula cream as it contains calendula plus other healing substances like aloe vera, avocado oil, and manuka honey. It's not usually in stores but you can easily get it online.

# DIARRHEA

## Quick Fix

**Activated charcoal** will often work, depending on the cause of the diarrhea. You can get it in capsule form in health food stores and drugstores. Inert and safe to take internally, it adsorbs toxins so effectively that it's used in emergency rooms for cases of poisoning or drug overdose.

Other options for quick relief include these remedies:

- **Arsenicum** for traveler's diarrhea and for diarrhea from food poisoning or bad water, often with a burning sensation and/or extreme weakness and fatigue yet restlessness.
- **Veratrum** for profuse, watery diarrhea with vomiting, abdominal cramps, and cold sweat.
- **Podophyllum** for "fire hydrant diarrhea." Got the picture?
- **Mercurius** for bloody or mucusy diarrhea, but if several doses in a day fail to clear up bloody diarrhea, please see your doctor.

## Ongoing Care

If diarrhea is caused by food poisoning, it usually goes away on its own after 24 hours. If it's caused by a virus, it can often be treated with one of the natural medicines above.

Activated charcoal should not be used longterm, as it can block the absorption of medicines and of nutrients from your food.

**China (Cinchona)** is a homeopathic medicine to take anytime you have lost fluids from diarrhea, vomiting, bleeding, etc.

## Preventing Recurrence

If you are traveling abroad, or camping, or have other reason to expect traveler's diarrhea or food poisoning, you can take a preventive dose of **Arsenicum** for each day of exposure.

If you have chronic recurring diarrhea, ask at your health food store for a good probiotic. If that still doesn't work, you may have irritable bowel syndrome. A holistic health professional (page 237) is likely to be able to treat it because there is often a strong mind-body component.

# EAR PROBLEMS

### Quick Fix for Water in Your Ears (Swimmer's Ear)

The homeopathic medicine **Kali mur.** (short for Kali muriaticum) is a special-order item to keep on hand if you or your child gets water in the ears frequently.

### Quick Fix for Ears Blocked in the Airplane

Blocked Eustachian tubes are a problem when you're about to get on an airplane because then the pressure cannot equalize when the cabin pressure is lowered. You can yawn, chew gum, or suck on something to keep the Eustachian tube open.

Try not to have a cold or fluid in your ears when you're about to fly. Use Kali mur. before you get on the plane if you have water in your ears from swimming or showering.

If you have a cold, use **Kali bic.**, the remedy for thick, sticky mucus that just won't budge, anywhere in the body. Get a 30c potency (strength), crush a few pellets, and dissolve them in a glass of water. Stir well and sip frequently before getting on the plane. If that doesn't work, it's safe to make a new cup of water on the plane, with the pellets that you remembered to take on the plane with you.

My clients frequently ask for help when they realize that they are about to get on a plane but their ears are blocked up. I've suggested Kali bic. (short for Kali bichromicum) and apparently it has often saved the day. Unlike Kali mur., Kali bic. is usually available in health food stores.

You can also open up your ear canal with this technique I learned from my chiropractic colleagues. It works by loosening up the mastoid bone behind the ears. You cup your hands over your ears, with your fingertips touching the bone behind your ears and spread equally around your ears. Pressing firmly on the bone, twist your hands backwards (clockwise with your left hand, counterclockwise with your right, if you imagine looking at your ear). Do this a couple of times as you breathe in, while your ears are trying to adjust to the pressure change.

# EARACHES AND EAR INFECTIONS

## Quick Fix

∽ **Mullein and garlic oil** from your local health food store.

Or the best-matching homeopathic medicine, for example:

∽ **Pulsatilla** for children who are clingy, needy and whiny when ill, although sweet, cuddly and affectionate when well. Thick yellow pus might be visible building up behind the eardrum.

∽ **Chamomilla** for children of a different temperament: the excruciating pain makes them act like brats, demanding things then throwing them down, demanding attention then telling you to go away, screaming inconsolably all the while. They might get an earache while teething; both ears might be red, or just one cheek might be red.

∽ **Belladonna** is another remedy for really painful ears with sudden onset and bright red cheeks. If kids are really sick they might have a high fever with heat radiating from the face, dilated pupils, and a tendency to mutter crazy talk.

## Ongoing Care

**Kali mur. 6x**, a cell salt, absorbs fluid from the middle ear.

Gently pulling on the ear can help to drain it. This works both during an ear infection and preventively. You hold the ear itself (not the ear lobe) and exert the gentlest of pressures outward and a little downward. It's safe for babies if you're really gentle. Try it for yourself, it feels good. Do it daily for kids who are prone to ear infections.

## Preventing Recurrence

The mothers in my health food store used to say simply "stop cow's milk." That single change was often enough to stop recurring ear infections. Breastfed babies are less likely to get ear infections. Eliminating other common allergens such as wheat, corn and eggs is also likely to help.

If not, the next thing to try (for babies and toddlers) would be an adjustment from a craniosacral therapist, chiropractor, or manipulating osteopath. Because of the position of the ears on a baby's head, the ear canal is more horizontal than an adult's and does not drain well, sometimes creating a susceptibility to infection. A gentle adjustment of the cranial bones can often fix the problem.

Treating ear infections with homeopathic medicines tends to break the cycle of recurrence because homeopathy supports the immune system. If none of these suggestions work, take your child (or yourself) to a professional homeopath, as homeopathy is especially good at shifting an overall pattern of illness.

## EMOTIONAL FIRST AID

### Quick Fix

∾ **Rescue Remedy** works for sudden frights or shocks of all kinds, and it can help heal physical traumas as well as emotional blows. It comes in a wide variety of formats now: a special blend for kids, another one for falling asleep at night, and the option of lozenges for those who want to avoid the few drops of alcohol in the original formula.

∾ **Ignatia** is a natural medicine for "hearing bad news": perhaps you just found out that a family member was in an accident or passed away suddenly. It's for stormy emotions of all kinds—sudden grief, rage, fright, betrayal, abandonment—when the person reacts with wild swings of emotion and a lot of sobbing. Perhaps someone finds out her husband has been cheating on her with her best friend, or a student is graded unfairly on an exam which might affect her college acceptances.

∾ **Gelsemium** is the medicine to use when the person reacts by going numb with shock, as if all the energy is drained out.

∾ Here's another tip: simply **taking some deep breaths** can help you calm down. You know how, when you get anxious, your chest tightens up and your breathing gets shallow? It works the other way around, too. Make yourself breathe deeply, and you'll feel calmer.

### Ongoing Care

Rescue Remedy is a blend of five of the 38 **flower essences,** all of which can be so helpful for different emotional states that they get their own chapter on page 160.

A **guided meditation CD** or a **yoga relaxation video.** If you practice yoga and/or meditation on a regular basis, you'll find yourself better prepared for the emotional ups and downs of life. Your yoga and meditation techniques will work better in an emergency if you've already "strengthened your inner muscles" by practicing them on a daily basis. More suggestions on pages 39–41.

## EYE PROBLEMS

**Blocked tear duct in an infant:** The homeopathic medicine **Silica** (safe for babies, see page 209).

**Foreign object in your eye:** **Aconite** (on the way to the ER, if needed).

**Black eye:** **Arnica** for the soft tissue bruising, **Symphytum** (the bone-mending remedy) for blows to the bone around the eye.

**Eyestrain** from too much computer use or reading fine print: The homeopathic medicine **Ruta grav.**, which can also work for floaters.

**Conjunctivitis: Breast milk.** For a baby, a little breast milk can act as a natural antibiotic. Otherwise try the best-matching homeopathic medicine:

- ∾ **Pulsatilla** is a common remedy for conjunctivitis and just about any condition in babies and small children, especially if they have the whiny-clingy-cuddly-affectionate nature and thick yellow pus-like discharge typical of children needing Pulsatilla.
- ∾ **Euphrasia,** a homeopathic medicine made from the herb Eyebright, works well for many conditions (conjunctivitis, allergies, colds) in which the eyes are red, itchy and watery, and the tears make the cheeks red and raw.
- ∾ **Graphites** if the eyelids are stuck together with crusty stuff.
- ∾ **Apis** if the eyelids look swollen, maybe warm and red, and if the discharge is like water rather than pus.

**Cataracts, glaucoma, and macular degeneration:** These chronic eye problems can be treated with nutritional supplements and homeopathic formulas available on the website of Dr. Edward Kondrot, **www.HealingTheEye.com** (click on the Vitamins tab). You'll also need the information in his book, *Ten Essentials to Save Your Sight.* Advanced cases require professional treatment at his clinic in Phoenix, Arizona.

# FATIGUE

## Quick Fix

"Double tall skinny vanilla." Only kidding!

The **Donna Eden Five-Minute Daily Energy Routine** is just that, and you can do it any time of the day—first thing in the morning, the mid-afternoon slump, the after-work crash. Open your meridians, massage your neurolymphatic points, and feel radiant in just five minutes. Check out the demo on GreenHealingTV on YouTube, or do a search for Donna Eden on YouTube and watch the queen of energy herself do a demo.

## Ongoing Care

Depends on why you are tired. Are you getting enough sleep? Tell me the truth. Really? If you're not asleep by 11 pm, do you get a second wind that keeps you awake for hours? In your case, the answer is to Tivo your late-night shows. Watching TV right before bed may disturb your sleep. Having electronic devices in your bedroom definitely does. Don't believe me? Get *Zapped* by Ann Louise Gittleman.

But what if you're tired because you are overworked, with too many responsibilities and not enough time? Maybe your adrenals are about to give up. They are the little glands on top of your kidneys that put out adrenaline in times of stress, which back in cave man days might have been occasionally, but nowadays is basically all the time.

Drinking coffee seems like a quick fix because it stimulates the adrenals to put out adrenaline, and then you feel that temporary buzz. But every time you use caffeine, it's like giving your adrenal glands a swift kick, and after a while they just roll over and play dead. Caffeine, by the way, is also found in guarana, soft drinks, and energy drinks.

If you can't get going in the morning without a cup of coffee, your adrenals are already in serious trouble. Human beings were not designed by evolution to need coffee in the morning. So here's what you do: Gradually switch to **Dandy Blend** instead of coffee. Dandy Blend is an amazingly delicious mocha-flavored hot drink mix which actually strengthens your liver. The homeopathic medicine **Chamomilla** may help if you feel cranky while getting off coffee.

Next, ask at your local health food store for an adrenal support formula such as Gaia Herb's Adrenal Health. Get those little adrenals back in shape with some great herbs like **licorice** and vitamins like **pantothenic acid** (Vitamin B5). Or support your adrenals and reduce your stress with the sacred Ayurvedic herb **holy basil**.

If you're not exercising every day, start now. You might think that exercising will make you feel more tired, but actually, it will get your circulation going and you'll feel better.

If you eat little or no animal foods, you may not have enough **B12**, which would definitely lead to tiredness. B12 is hard to absorb in the stomach, which is why it's traditionally been given by injection. Now it's available as lozenges so that it will absorb under the tongue.

Women who are exhausted and overworked plus having hormonal symptoms, including weepiness and irritability with loved ones and feeling "at the end of your rope" can safely try the homeopathic medicine **Sepia 6c** once a day for a month. If it matches your symptoms well, you'll see why my clients call it "the vacation in a bottle."

Or take a homeopathic combination such as Heel's Exhaustion.

These supplements will give you enough energy to investigate more deeply into the causes of your fatigue. It might be your thyroid gland, for example. You could read one of these books for tests you can do, supplements you can take, and dietary changes you can make to have more energy:

∾ Dr. Datis Kharrazian's *Why Do I Still Have Thyroid Symptoms When My Lab Tests Are Normal?*
∾ Dr. Jacob Teitelbaum's *Feeling Fat, Fuzzy or Frazzled?*
∾ Dr. Mark Hyman's *UltraMetabolism*.

Depending on how serious your situation is, you may be able to turn it around with the help of these books, or you may need the guidance of a holistic health care professional. In the meantime, make yourself a fabulous mocha frappe with Dandy Blend, cocoa powder, and coconut milk.

## FIRST AID

For any serious injury, call 9-1-1 first, then give the following homeopathic medicines while waiting for the ambulance. Homeopathy is
especially useful in these situations because it can work so fast. Give the
medicines in water to make them stronger (page 207–208).

- Bleeding: **Phosphorus** (page 197).
- Broken bones: Give frequent doses of **Arnica** on the spot to reduce
  pain and swelling while waiting for emergency medical care (page
  182). Once the bone is set, give **Symphytum** once a day and **Calc.
  phos. 6x** twice a day (page 173) to help the bone mend faster.
- Bruising, blows to the head: **Arnica**. If your child plays a sport
  which involves blows to the head, please be very, very careful, as
  blows to the head can cause tissue damage to the brain which does
  not show up on an X-ray. Protect your child with a good helmet,
  good safety instructions, and Arnica to take immediately after any
  head injury.
- Burns: **Aloe** (page 158), **Calendula** (page 186)
- Cuts, scrapes, abrasions, lacerations: **Calendula** (page 186)
- Electrical shock or burn: **Phosphorus** (page 197)
- Heat exhaustion, heat cramps, dehydration: **Belladonna** and the
  tissue salt **Nat. mur. 6x** (page 172)
- Hit your finger with a hammer: **Hypericum** (page 191)
- Shock or fright from a potentially fatal accident: **Aconite**

If you are likely to encounter these situations (maybe you lead
wilderness expeditions? or have a large family of rambunctious kids
in a remote rural area?) I recommend Eileen Naumann's *Help! and
Homeopathy: What to Do in an Emergency Before 911 Arrives*. It has lots
of practical information about safely handling dozens of emergencies,
including serious medical emergencies.

# FLU

## Quick Fix

If you catch it right in the beginning, **"Oscillo"** may stave it off. (This is the nickname for Oscillococcinum, and nobody else can pronounce it either.) Get it before flu season so you have it on hand. Any health food store and many drug stores will have it. You don't need a whole tube at once, though, just a few pellets.

## Ongoing Care

Once a flu gets going, it may be too late for "Oscillo." You'll get the best results with one of the following medicines, the one that matches your symptoms. Also take a good herbal immune or wellness formula such as Zand's Insure Formula, plus **elderberry syrup** (page 158).

- **Gelsemium** is the most common medicine for the flu and other viral conditions. You can recognize someone who needs it— drooping eyelids, so tired they can't get out of bed, they have fever and chills, and they feel apathetic, unlike our next contender...

- **Arsenicum** is for people who are extremely tired (like Gelsemium), but they are likely to be anxious and fretful, restless and uncomfortable in bed. They are especially likely to be awake and restless between midnight and 2 am, their worst time. They are likely to have a sore throat and a drippy, watery nasal discharge. They might also have digestive symptoms, but a more likely remedy for a flu with digestive symptoms is...

- **Nux vomica.** Doesn't the name just sound like it's for vomiting? Big clue—it's a great remedy for the digestive system, from beginning (heartburn) to end (hemorrhoids). Use it for the flu when the person has the chills and is really sensitive to noise and to being disturbed (they are really irritable). They can't stand the slightest draft of cold air that creeps in under the covers, where they will stay all bundled up.

- **Rhus tox.**, used mostly for little blistery conditions like poison ivy and cold sores, can be used for the flu when accompanied by cold sores, plus the person is likely to have joint pain and to feel worse in damp weather, better with a hot bath.

Many other possible natural medicines for the flu are described in Randall Neustaedter's *Flu: Alternative Treatments and Prevention.* It's worth taking the time to figure out your best-matching flu medicine because It's likely to be the same every time you get the flu. Having it on hand could save you a lot of time lost from work.

## Preventing Recurrence

"Oscillo," the top selling flu remedy in France, also works great for prevention. For some people, and for some season's flu viruses, **Influenzinum** works better. It may be a little harder to find in stores but you can usually get it from Homeopathic Educational Services, www.Homeopathic.com, and Washington Homeopathics, www. HomeopathyWorks.com.

Usually a 9c (low potency) of Influenzinum is used for prevention and 30c to treat an actual flu. Oscillo only comes in one potency.

**Dosage:** when the flu season starts, take either remedy once a week for four weeks, then once a month for the remainder of the flu season.

Take an additional preventive dose every day that you are directly and closely exposed to someone with the flu, in your family or at work.

When you're feeling rundown and likely to get sick, take the "nip it in the bud" remedy **Ferrum phos.** (page 170). Also take these early warning symptoms as a sign that you need to slow down and take care of yourself. This is especially true for moms who tend to care for everyone else first. But if you get sick, who will take care of them? So be sure to get enough rest, eat healthy food, and minimize coffee and sugar. This is a great time to take your immune-boosting formula.

# GAS (INTESTINAL)

**Quick Fix**

- **Activated charcoal** can absorb many times its volume in gas. You can get activated charcoal caps at your health food store. Spoiler alert: they will turn your poop black. But they are a safe way to absorb the occasional gas attack. They can't be used routinely as they block the absorption of nutrients and oral medications.
- **Peppermint oil** is a natural dispeller of gas. Look for "enteric-coated" capsules, ones that are coated to survive the stomach acid and make their way down into the intestines where the problem arises.

**Ongoing Care**

The homeopathic medicine that matches your symptoms can take care of your gas problem and most likely rebalance other digestive issues at the same time. The most common:

- **Argentum nitricum** for loud, rumbling, embarrassing gas, in a person who may be very anxious ("what if this happens? what if that happens?") and who may also have intense sweet cravings but feel worse after eating sweets.
- **China (Cinchona)** for people who may also have a lot of rumbling and gurgling, maybe with a feeling of fermenting, perhaps after eating spoiled meat; perhaps with weakness, feeling drained and exhausted.
- **Lycopodium** for people who feel full after just a couple of bites and who need to loosen their belts after eating; "lower down" gas (in other words, they are more likely to pass gas than to burp).
- **Carbo veg.**, interestingly, is made from charcoal. The person is more likely to burp than to pass gas. They may be exhausted and have "air hunger," a feeling of not getting enough oxygen.

## Preventing Recurrence

Why is your body producing gas? It could be because you aren't digesting your food properly, in which case there are multiple possible approaches:

- Take supplemental **digestive enzymes** such as ReNew Life's Digest-More, an excellent brand made from raw plant enzymes.
- If you prefer **herbal tea**, try a blend such as Yogi Tea Stomach Ease Tea or Lemon Ginger Tea, or make your own blend with peppermint, which is a traditional digestive aid.
- Eat **raw foods**, which will provide enzymes your body can use to make its own digestive enzymes.
- Eat foods that are "predigested," for example traditional **fermented foods** like kefir, miso, and fresh sauerkraut.
- Eat simpler meals so that your body does not have to digest protein (which requires an acidic environment) and carbohydrates (which require an alkaline environment) at the same time. Eat these two types of food separately.
- Or perhaps you need better intestinal flora. In this case you need a good blend of **probiotics** such as Klaire Ther-Biotic, MegaFood's MegaFlora or Jarro-dophilus. Look for a probiotic that contains billions, not just millions, of organisms per capsule.

# GOUT

## Quick Fix

You'll have to order these remedies ahead of time so you have them on hand for a painful gout attack.

- **Colchicum** is the best homeopathic remedy for gout, and you should put it in water and succuss it to make it stronger (page 208) because the pain of gout is so excruciating.
- **Urtica urens** (nettle) tincture apparently works by dissolving uric acid crystals in the joints and passing them out through the urine. Or at least gout sufferers report feeling better while their pee looks darker. Put a dropperful of the tincture in a cup of water or juice and sip on it occasionally to use it up over an 8 hour period, repeating as needed in an acute attack.

The following remedies from your health food store can tide you over while you're waiting for your Colchicum and Urtica urens:

- **Belladonna** if the joint is swollen, bright red, hot to the touch, perhaps with sudden-onset pain throbbing like a pulse.
- **Bryonia** if the pain is worse from the slightest movement or jarring motion. The person is grouchy and irritable from the pain. If you bump into their painful joint by mistake, look out!
- **Stinging nettle** (Urtica dioica) instead of Urtica urens.

## Ongoing Care

Gout is caused by a combination of dietary factors (too much fatty foods and alcohol) and the body's inability to clear the resulting uric acid. In addition to the food suggestions in Part One:

- Focus on **cherries and cherry juice** when it comes to fruit.
- Emphasize **fish and fish oils** instead of red meat.
- Tweak your supplements by adding **Vitamin C** and the anti-inflammatories **quercetin and bromelain.**
- **Detox your liver** (which has been struggling to keep up with all your past fatty foods and alcohol) and strengthen your kidneys (**Gaia Herb's Liver Support** and **uva ursi/corn silk tea** for your kidneys).

## HAIR, THINNING OR GRAYING

No quick fix here, but these suggestions are safe and inexpensive. I have seen results in my women customers and clients, although I have never had occasion to try them with men.

### Graying Hair

PABA (para-amino benzoic acid), one of the B vitamins, has darkened gray hair in some research studies, and I've seen it with my own eyes with some of my customers. Before you get too excited, let me say that the research studies have been mixed and that the effect wears off two months after taking it. Also the most consistent results have come from taking a *lot* of PABA (many grams a day), which can throw your other B vitamins out of whack, so you should take a strong B-complex at the same time.

The larger question is why some people have a symptom (gray hair) which seems to be associated with a nutritional deficiency. Because of the "biochemic individuality" associated with the need for nutrients, these people may have a genetic tendency to need much more PABA than other people.

Unless you have a holistic health care professional who is monitoring your extremely high use of one vitamin, I don't think it's safe to keep taking that much PABA indefinitely. The best results in the research studies, apparently, came from people who had been prescribed high doses of PABA for other reasons.

The customers in my store who got results were able to do it with a minor addition of a gram or two of PABA, which would be two to four of the typical 500 milligram caps. Worth a try and safe if you take a B complex with it.

### Thinning Hair

Restoring thinning hair depends on the underlying cause: hormonal imbalance (in women), or the lack of nutrients needed for strong hair. Neither of these reasons would explain male pattern baldness (sorry, guys).

**Hormone balancing for women:** These remedies have worked well in my practice for women with thinning hair during a time of hormonal change like pregnancy, post-partum, perimenopause or menopause:

- **Sepia** has worked well for women who are overwhelmed, exhausted, at the end of their rope, with weepiness at the drop of a hat and irritability with their loved ones. These women may have a sluggish circulation and dark brown menstrual blood. They are likely to feel better from vigorous exercise because it gets their circulation going. They may feel so drained that they wish they could just get away from it all, but if they take a vacation, they're just as tired afterwards.
- **Lachesis** works well for quite a different type, women who have intense energy rising up inside them. They need to discharge the energy to get relief, and this discharge may take the form of hot flashes or of a verbal outburst. They can be passionate, jealous, and sometimes cruel when they lash out at others.

These are the most common remedies for hormonal hair loss. A professional homeopath can help if these don't match, and your other hormonal symptoms are likely to get better at the same time.

**Nutritional deficiencies:** Weak, thin, brittle hair that falls out by the handfuls can indicate a lack of the nutrients needed to create healthy hair, such as **biotin** (one of the B vitamins) and **cysteine** (one of the amino acids). An easy way to get all the nutrients you need is a combination formula like **MegaFoods' Skin, Nails and Hair Formula.**

If you tend to have weak, brittle nails and skin that's slow to heal as well as thinning hair, I would take the cell salt **Silicea** (page 178).

Or you can take the mineral silica as **Bio-Sil,** a highly concentrated, highly absorbable form. It allows the body to make its own collagen, which is essential for youthful, healthy skin, hair and joints.

**Jojoba oil** rubbed into the scalp can also provide needed nutrients. Rub it in at night, put a towel on your pillow, wash it out in the morning.

**Egg yolks** are a rich source of cysteine, which is why egg yolks are a home remedy for thinning hair. If you have extra egg yolks anyway (for example you're on a diet that only allows egg whites), you could have fun making your own hair conditioner with egg yolks and cider vinegar.

**Do you really have thinning hair?** When women come to see me for thinning hair, I always think their hair looks fine. "See?" they say, "See? There's nothing left," and meanwhile I'm looking at this beautiful thick hair. Sometimes I think they need a remedy for feeling badly about how they look, which is an unfortunate effect of the unrealistic portrayal of women in our media.

---

### THE VANISHING DARK CIRCLES

Speaking of women feeling badly about how they look, a young woman consulted me recently for dark circles under her eyes. She looked fine to me! This lovely young woman seemed totally obsessed with non-existent dark circles.

I gave her the remedy **Nat. mur.**, because it can help with dark circles — and with feeling that you look terrible. In fact it's also remedy for hair loss after a typical Nat. mur. event, silent grief ("I never shed a tear").

People who need Nat. mur. tend to be very self-critical because deep down they believe they lost a loved one because they weren't good enough. "If only I were perfect," they believe on a subconscious, irrational level, "he never would have left me." Trying to protect themselves against further loss, they may scrutinize themselves for any imperfection and over-focus on details like thinning hair or dark circles under their eyes.

# HEMORRHOIDS

## Quick Fix

Witch hazel (a traditional astringent available in any drug store), applied externally to shrink hemorrhoids.

Or if you can get these products quickly, they are likely to work faster than witch hazel because they are stronger: Avenoc Hemorrhoid Cream or Nelson's Hemorrhoid Cream.

## Ongoing and Preventive Care

This depends on why you have hemorrhoids, which are basically varicose veins of the anus. Here are some possible causes and their remedies.

**Straining to have a bowel movement?** This straining action can make those veins in the rectum pop out. The solution is to treat the constipation (see page 75).

**Do you have varicose veins in your legs?** If the basic problem is weakness in the walls of your blood vessels, leading to sagging of the veins and pooling of the circulation, you can strengthen the walls of the blood vessels as follows:

ᴖ  Calc. fluor. 6x, the cell salt (page 173)

ᴖ  Rutin and bioflavonoids (page 65)

**Are the hemorrhoids hormonal?** Did they come out during pregnancy or labor? or during menopause or perimenopause? If so, take Sepia 6c daily ongoing, or Sepia 30c short term if the symptoms are intense (see page 204 for more instructions), in addition to the recommendations for varicose veins above.

**Is your liver congested?** The blood flowing through these veins in the rectum would normally flow through the liver on its way back to the heart, but if the liver is backed up, the circulation will also back up, like a great big traffic jam. Cirrhosis of the liver would be an extreme example of shutting down circulation through it. But circulation can also be slowed as the liver struggles to keep up with its job of breaking down all the toxins that enter our body from this overly chemicalized world. Solutions include:

∾ **Castor oil packs** (page 79) on the liver.

∾ An herbal **liver cleanse** (your local health food store will have a good blend).

∾ The homeopathic medicines **Nux vomica** and **Sulphur** on alternate days

## HERPES AND SHINGLES

**Quick Fix**

- For both cold sores (oral herpes) and genital herpes, **lysine** applied topically (for example Quantum Super Lysine Plus) and also lysine capsules taken internally (two 500mg capsules, three times a day) will often dry up herpes lesions quickly.
- **Red marine algae** works both to prevent and to cure, both orally and topically. Take 2500 mg a day (it may be labeled Gigartina). You can even pull apart a capsule and sprinkle it on the herpes lesion.
- Olive leaf extract is also highly effective against the herpes virus.

**Ongoing Care**

Use the universal immune-supporting supplements like Vitamin C, probiotics, and echinacea. Add these products specifically for herpes:

- **Zinc**, especially good for healing any skin problem.
- **Lomatium**, a wonderful antiviral herb.
- **Propolis**, the amazing substance that bees, in their wisdom, use to keep their hive a totally sterile environment. Use topically for cold sores and genital herpes.

If you always get herpes before your period, you are probably getting other hormonal symptoms and would benefit from an overall hormone balancing regimen (see page 104).

Or consider whether your herpes outbreaks represent a larger picture of physical or emotional stress for you. If so, homeopathic medicines may offer the best all-around solution. For example:

- **Nat. mur.** is the most common homeopathic medicine for cold sores, in my experience. See the description under **Canker Sores.** The cold sores may come on after sun exposure, after a cold or flu, or in someone in a longterm suppressed grief state. The eruption is likely to have a blister filled with a clear fluid.
- **Rhus tox.:** the eruption may come on while you have the flu, and/ or it looks like a little bunch of tiny blisters which may be really

itchy. It looks and itches like poison ivy.

∾ **Hepar sulph.:** when you're feeling really sensitive and irritable, and the lesion itself is really sensitive to cold or to touch.

∾ **Graphites:** when the sore exudes a honey-colored fluid which then dries and crusts over. Often needed in menopausal women.

Directions on pages 204–208 for these remedies.

## Preventing Recurrence

If you get herpes frequently or if you are going through a phase when you feel extra susceptible, you may benefit from taking 1000mg a day of **red marine algae (Gigartina)**.

Or take one 500 mg capsule of **lysine** daily. Take additional capsules at the very first tingle before an outbreak (for a total of two caps three times a day). Lysine is an amino acid that competes with the amino acid arginine, which is the favorite food for the herpes virus.

Then again, you could avoid the arginine-containing foods, which are easy to remember: think Reese's peanut butter cups. In other words, avoid chocolate and nuts, especially peanut butter. Arginine is also in muscle-building protein powders.

Finally, avoid the stressors that bring on herpes for you. Some people get cold sores when they get colds or go out in the sun, but most people get herpes under emotional stress. Try to keep calm (deep breathing, yoga, quit your job) and when you're extra tense, take extra lysine.

## Shingles

These painful or itchy blisters are a form of herpes and may respond to **lysine** internally and externally. Follow the other supplement recommendations for herpes. In terms of homeopathic remedies, **Traumeel** in liquid form, taken orally, can get the body out of its crisis/trauma mode, then apply Traumeel in ointment form (applied around the area of the shingles blisters, not on top of it).

## HORMONE BALANCING FOR WOMEN

### Quick Fix

Try the homeopathic combination remedies aimed at women's hormonal issues just to get you started while you follow the suggestions below. For example: Hyland's PMS, Menstrual Cramps or Menopause; or Boiron's Cyclease PMS or Cyclease Cramp.

### Ongoing Care

Why is this such a big issue for Western women? We seem to suffer hormonal symptoms unlike women in traditional societies and women eating a more traditional diet. There are many factors in our toxic world, including endocrine-disrupting chemicals, and in our unnatural diet, including an unhealthy balance of essential fatty acids.

We can create a beneficial hormonal balance without needing either hormone replacement therapy or bio-identical hormones. We just need to give our bodies the blueprint (via a homeopathic medicine) and the building blocks to implement it (with herbs, supplements, and a natural diet). We also need to eliminate the factors in our environment that can disrupt our hormones.

Here are some things to do for starters:

**Take essential fatty acids** such as Nordic Naturals Ultimate Omega or Barlean's Omega Swirl for Women. Eat foods that are good sources of essential fatty acids (coldwater fish plus the tiny precious seeds — flax seeds, hemp seeds, chia seeds, borage oil). Eliminate foods with toxic fats, like commercial cookies, crackers, cereals, and other products that are made to sit on the shelf.

**Use herbs** that women have used since time immemorial to create hormonal balance, now blended for your convenience: herbs such as dong quai, licorice, burdock, motherwort and wild yam in Vitanica's Women's Phase formulas. Black cohosh and maca are two other herbs widely used for women's hormonal conditions.

**Find the best-matching homeopathic medicine**, ideally by working with a professional homeopath, but if that is not an option, get Eileen Nauman's *Beauty in Bloom* and Catherine Coulter's *Nature and Human Personality* to try to find your individual medicine. *Beauty in Bloom* also has lots of practical advice for natural healing during menopause.

**Eliminate chemicals** as much as possible from your bodycare products, household cleaners, detergents, pesticides, lawn and garden products, and other items like air fresheners and drier sheets. Some of these products contain endocrine disrupters. New sources of toxicity are being discovered all the time. Why take a chance? Keep checking the Environmental Working Group website, **www.EWG.org**. This change will benefit your whole family and support your health in many ways like preventing cancer, not just protecting your hormones. Learn lots of practical tips for a chemical-free household from *The Non-Toxic Avenger* by Deanna Duke.

If these do-it-yourself suggestions are not sufficient to relieve your symptoms, I would go to a naturopathic doctor or functional medicine doctor (pages 237–238). They can do saliva testing for your hormone levels and create a protocol for you based on the results.

Or go to a professional homeopath (pages 238–239) who can find your best-matching homeopathic medicine like fitting you for a custom-tailored suit. You will still need good essential fatty acids and other nutritional support, though.

A homeopathic remedy can help balance your hormones not by bringing in hormones or hormone-like substances from the outside (whether synthetic or bio-identical or herbal) but by reminding your body how to find the balance it naturally has. The remedy provides the information, the blueprint, the template. It's like repairing a building by going back to the original architect's drawings. Your body will still need the right building blocks (nutrients) to implement the plan.

# INSOMNIA

## Quick Fix

∾ **5-HTP** helps the body create serotonin, so not only does it help with sleep, it also helps with depression, stress, carbohydrate cravings, and many other plagues of our modern lifestyle. For example, try Natural Factors' Stress-Relax 5-HTP.

∾ **Calms Forte** is a blend of cell salts and herbs traditionally used to induce sleep (see page 175 for more on cell salts). You could keep it by your bed and dissolve a couple in your mouth when going to bed, then a couple more if you wake up and can't get back to sleep.

∾ **Melatonin** is the sleep hormone, available as a supplement, although it's better to encourage your body to make its own (see the discussion of blue light on the next page).

## Ongoing Care

Herbal blends such as **Gaia Herb's Sound Sleep, Vitanica Sleep Blend**.

Homeopathic medicines for insomnia are useful because they tend to address the underlying reason. For example:

∾ **Coffea** for "insomnia from joy," like a bride the night before her wedding, or someone on the eve of a special vacation or joyful family reunion. Also may be useful for kids who are "tired and wired." You know how kids can get more and more wound up at night and overstimulate themselves having fun.

∾ **Ignatia**, the "rehearsal remedy," for people who lie awake brooding over an upsetting situation or a relationship problem, reviewing what they said or might have said differently or practicing what they might say the next time.

∾ **Arsenicum** for the worry wart who tends to be awake from midnight to 2 am, restless and fretful, perhaps moving from one bed to another in the hopes of getting more comfortable, but really awake because of anxieties about practical things (money, health, job situation, fantasizing about being on the brink of homelessness).

~ **Nux vomica** for people who have liver problems because they eat too much fatty food and/or drink too much alcohol. They may also be hard-working, hard-driving, ambitious business people who overuse stimulants to get ahead. Typically they would wake up around 3 or 4 am and lie awake planning their next business strategy or get-rich-quick scheme.

~ **Lycopodium** may work for people who have liver problems leading to low blood sugar, which means that they "sleep eat." I had such a client once. She knew she was sleep-eating because she would wake up in the morning with the cookie drawer open in the kitchen and her bed full of cookie crumbs. Lycopodium helped, but so did having some protein in the evening to keep her blood sugar level from plummeting while she slept.

## Lifestyle Support

Avoid using electronics for a couple of hours before bed so that you can settle your mind, and also to avoid electromagnetic field exposure. If you absolutely must use the computer before bed (*finally* got the kids down), use blue-light blocking glasses, which you can get online. Computer monitors emit blue light, which makes your pineal gland think you're looking at the blue sky, and hey, it's time to play. Then the pineal gland doesn't make melatonin, the sleep hormone, which is part of the pineal's job description.

You also need to minimize electronics in your bedroom because of the EMF exposure. Please get Ann Louise Gittleman's *Zapped* and she will lead you through an electronics census of each room in your house (baby monitors, dimmer switches, cell phone chargers, oh my!) then provide practical suggestions for minimizing exposure.

Speaking of electronics, please also avoid falling asleep with the TV on, especially the TV news. All that frightening and shocking stuff, which they play on purpose to get you hooked on the TV news, will seep into your brain without your conscious mind being able to filter it, which can disturb your sleep.

# KIDNEY STONES

## Quick Fix

If you're reading this and you have a kidney stone on its way out, it's too late. Or maybe not. You could take a homeopathic medicine on the way to the emergency room. If you can relax the ureter so it doesn't go into spasm from the pain, it just might let that sucker go. If you have **Mag. phos.** on hand—the medicine for muscle cramps and spasms—take a few pellets right away, then put a few into a small water bottle, shake well and sip frequently.

## Ongoing Care

The rainforest herb **chanca piedra** has traditionally been used for breaking up kidney stones and gallstones, with this use recently backed by research. Reportedly chanca piedra can dissolve the stones in one to two weeks. I have several cases among my own clients of before-and-after ultrasounds indicating that stones were dissolved. It is inexpensive, safe (except for pregnant women and people on diuretics or medications for diabetes), and worth a try.

## Preventing Recurrence

**Chanca piedra** can also work preventively for people with a tendency to form kidney stones. It also helps if you reduce meat consumption, avoid oxalate-containing foods (chard, spinach, peanuts, chocolate, black tea), drink a lot of water, and take extra **magnesium** such as Natural Calm.

## Take Your Remedy Kit to the ER

Recently I had an attack of intense, sudden onset abdominal pain. It wasn't clear what caused it, so I headed for the ER with my homeopathic emergency kit in hand. The doctor who examined me was pretty certain it was a kidney stone but sent me for a CAT scan to be sure. While I waited . . . and waited . . . and waited, I took multiple doses of a remedy. The CAT scan showed that in fact I had just had a kidney stone— but it was already gone!

Of course I'll never know if the remedy had anything to do with it. This story is meant to reflect on the appropriate uses of conventional and alternative healing.

## MENOPAUSE SYMPTOMS

**Quick Fixes**

- For hot flashes: **Deep abdominal breathing.** Slowing the breath to 6 to 8 breaths per minute instead of the usual 15 or more seems to shift the body's thermoregulation system. To learn how, lie on your back with a hand on your stomach so that you can feel your abdomen rising as you push your diaphragm down to breathe in. It's easier if you start with the exhale: squeeze every last bit of air out of your lungs, squeezing up with your diaphragm like making a tight fist under your ribs. Then reverse it to breathe in, and your abdomen will naturally rise. Once you've got the hang of it, you can do it anywhere.

- For vaginal dryness: Apply **coconut oil** or **liquid vitamin E.**

- For heart palpitations: These are common during menopause and are no cause for alarm (unless you also have symptoms of a possible heart attack such as shortness of breath, dizziness, fainting, and nausea; women often don't experience chest pain or pressure during a heart attack). Be sure to take **magnesium** and **CoQ10** and add the heart tonic **hawthorn** (see page 158).

- Insomnia is covered in its own section.

**Ongoing Care**

Herbs can provide natural hormonal balance. **Black cohosh** works for some women, **red clover** for others, and blends of herbs generally work best, such as Vitanica Women's Phase II. Estroven, a popular brand of black cohosh, blends it with calcium and B vitamins, while Promensil is a recommended brand of red clover because it has guaranteed levels of the active ingredients (a major concern with herbal supplements).

**Maca** is another herb that works well for menopausal and post-menopausal symptoms like hot flashes, night sweats, mood swings, vaginal dryness and fatigue.

Be sure to get enough **essential fatty acids:** Nordic Naturals Omega Woman or Barlean's Omega Swirl for Women.

A homeopathic remedy that matches your symptoms can help a lot, for example:

- **Sepia** is the most frequently used in my practice, for women who are exhausted, overworked, with no time for themselves, perhaps weepy or irritable with their loved ones, feeling draggy, and maybe even feeling their uterus or bladder literally dragging down. It can help hot flashes, insomnia, heart palpitations, and "hormonal brain fog" (when you feel like information just goes in one ear and out the other). Sepia can be used for any hormonal time (PMS, menses, pregnancy, postpartum, perimenopause or menopause) in a 6c strength for daily use or a 30c strength for occasional use. It's available in any health food store.

- **Lachesis** has a motto: "pent-up energy looking for a discharge," which can come in the form of hot flashes or verbal outbursts. (One of my clients who needed Lachesis said about herself, "I use my tongue like a stun gun.") Miranda Castro does a wonderful impersonation of Lachesis on the GreenHealingTV channel on YouTube: search for Hot Flashes.

- **Cimicifuga** is for menopause, PMS, or other time of hormonal flux when you feel like there's a "black cloud over your head" or your mood swings are so intense that you feel like you're going crazy.

More about how to use homeopathics on pages 204–208.

## Lifestyle Support

Guided imagery actually worked for hot flashes in a small study conducted at a university hospital in Sweden, in which six women met once a week for 12 weeks for an hour of group relaxation—and had their hot flashes reduced by almost 75%, while reducing other menopausal symptoms and increasing feelings of well-being. Relax with Belleruth Naparstek's lovely guided meditation CD, *Mastering Menopause*.

Women in other cultures who eat traditional foods don't suffer from menopause symptoms the way American women do. One reason could be the quality of fats in our diet. We need good essential fatty acids as the building blocks for a good hormonal balance. They're hard to get; we need to incorporate fish, fish oils and/or flax, hemp, and other oil-bearing seeds. The foods that destroy these fats are easy to come by: junk foods, deep-fried foods, baked goods, and any processed foods that are meant to sit on the shelf for months. The food industry has figured out how to replace trans fats with new bad fats that don't show up on the label. (Another good reason to avoid foods with labels, and to take supplemental essential fatty acids unless you are a paragon of virtue in the healthy food department.)

Soy foods seem to be controversial these days. However, tradition-ally-prepared soy foods (including tofu and soymilk) have been part of the Asian diet for centuries, and women in those countries don't get hormonal symptoms, hypothyroidism, or reproductive cancers like we do. Asians' rates of chronic disease increase sharply when they adopt a Western diet.

I would avoid *processed* soy foods like fake meats and the isolated soy protein powder added to meal replacement bars. (These bars don't replace food in any case. Our bodies need real food that looks like it came out of the ground or off a tree, not these fake foods labeled 'meal replacement' to fool us). Women with estrogen-dependent cancers should also avoid soy because it has estrogen-like qualities.

# MENSTRUAL CRAMPS

**Quick Fix**

The easiest approach is to use a homeopathic combination remedy such as **Hyland's Menstrual Cramps** or **Boiron Cyclease Cramp Tablets.**

If you can think a bit despite the pain, your individualized remedy will help you in other ways. For example:

- **Sepia** for women who feel like their uterus is going to just slide down and out, who get totally exhausted and brain-dead, weepy at the drop of a hat, irritable with their loved ones, and who crave chocolate (or pickles) and feel better when they get their circulation going with vigorous exercise. Sepia is more likely to work for older women, whereas young girls might try . . .

- **Pulsatilla** for "changeable symptoms": this can include the fluctuating moods of a teenager or the changeable quality of the menstrual flow itself, which can stop and start a few times each month.

- **Lilium tigrinum** is for women with the same "bearing down sensation" as Sepia except— big difference!— they have a high libido whereas the Sepia woman's libido is long gone.

- **Mag. phos.** and **Colocynth** are for women whose cramps feel better when they pull their knees up to their chest (maybe pressing a book or pillow into their abdomen) and/or use a heating pad. They are similar except if forced to choose, women who need Mag. phos. would choose warmth and women who need Colocynth would choose pressure. Also Colocynth is much more likely to match if the woman has experienced injustice or suppressed anger.

- **Cimicifuga** is for menstrual cramps that feel like they are shooting across the abdomen, sometimes accompanied by a stiff or sore neck. It's for women who have a "black cloud over their head" and mood swings so bad, they say they feel like they are going crazy.

- **Chamomilla** is for women whose menstrual cramps are so intense, they feel like they are going into labor. The intense pain makes the woman so crabby, she keeps demanding things then rejecting them. Chamomilla may bring peace to the household.

You can also use this simple **Reflex Technique** for menstrual cramps. Coming from the chiropractic specialty Sacro-Occipital Technique, it can work quickly for many women by establishing a circuit with the reflex point for the uterus.

∾ First you "hug" yourself only with your left arm, putting your left hand high up on your right lower neck.

∾ Next, find the middle of your pubic bone with your right hand. Bring your hand up towards your abdomen until your fingers slide just off the bone, then move about an inch to the right. Feel around this area for a tender spot.

∾ With your right hand, rub counter-clockwise four to six times. Repeat hourly until symptoms are alleviated.

### Ongoing Care
Essential fatty acids, hormone-balancing herbs, and extra magnesium (to prevent cramps) will help a lot.

### Lifestyle Support
Exercise will help everyone, not just the Sepia-type woman. When I was in high school, our gym teacher made us do situps—the last thing in the world you want to do when you have cramps, but they worked right away.

# MIGRAINES

## Quick Fix

Try **Migrastick**, a roller stick with essential oils of lavender and peppermint which you apply to your temples, forehead, and neck. Essential oils work really fast because when you inhale them through your nose, they touch receptor cells which directly connect with a deep part of your brain. Just one long nerve cell connects your nose and your brain, and it's the most direct port of entry into your brain.

## Ongoing Care

The herbs **butterbur** and **feverfew** work to prevent migraines. Butterbur is actually recommended by American Headache Academy doctors. Rainbow Light's Migrasolve Petadolex contains butterbur and riboflavin (vitamin B2), which also works preventively. Gaia Herbs' Migraprofen includes feverfew plus stress-relief herbs like skullcap, valerian, and kava kava. Feverfew may even work to treat the migraine once it's already underway.

Preventive herbs work best when taken daily, but they should do their job within a few months, and taking them daily longterm may not be safe. Also feverfew is not recommended for pregnant or nursing women.

You can also try taking **magnesium**, especially if you have other indications (like muscle cramps) that your magnesium is low.

You probably already know that it may help to lie down in a dark room. How about doing some **deep belly breathing** (described under **Hot Flashes**) or progressive relaxation while you are there? You might even put a cold pack behind your neck and a hot pack on your feet to draw the congested circulation away from your head.

## Lifestyle Support

There are many ways to break the cycle of recurring migraines because there are many possible causes. The best summary I've seen is on Dr. Mark Hyman's blog. Go to **www.DrMarkHyman.com**, then to his blog, and search for "how to end migraines."

# MUSCLE CRAMPS

**Quick Fix**

∾ For calf cramps: grab the toes and pull up towards the top of the foot to stretch the calf. This usually works right away.

∾ For muscle cramps in general: **Mag. phos. 30c.**

∾ For cramps in the digestive system (stomach cramps or cramping in the colon):

  o **Nux vomica** if the person matches the Nux vomica type (workaholic, ambitious, competitive, money-oriented, stimulating himself to work long hours at his business by using stimulants like coffee, cigarettes, drugs both medicinal and possibly recreational, and spicy, fatty junk food).

  o **Ignatia** if the person matches the Ignatia type (the cramps are likely to be psychosomatic and associated with emotional upset).

For menstrual cramps, see that section.

**Ongoing Care**

Take extra magnesium because muscle cramps are often due to a magnesium deficiency.

# NAILS: CRACKED, SPLIT, OR FUNGAL

### Quick Fix

Thuja can be used as a toenail dip for fungus under the nails. Dissolve a pellet of the homeopathic remedy in about half a cup of water (you may have to crush it to dissolve it) and put it in a clean container like a deli container. Soak your toenails in it for ten minutes twice a day. My clients have told me they can see clean pink nails growing out within the first week. This seems biologically impossible to me but a number of clients have told me the same thing.

The cell salt Silicea (see page 178) can strengthen brittle or soft nails. I use it myself and I can feel the ends of my nails get hard within a few days. This is definitely biologically impossible, since it takes weeks for nails to grow out from the nail bed, but it works for me every time.

### Ongoing Care

Strong healthy nails need specific amino acids (elements of protein), vitamins and minerals. Healthy skin and hair need the same nutrients. You can get them in a blend, for example **MegaFoods' Skin, Nails and Hair Formula.**

You can also get the vitamins and minerals from herbal blends like **Gaia Herb's Hair, Skin & Nail Support.** For example, silica is an essential mineral for strengthening nails, and herbs like horsetail are rich sources of silica. Taking the homeopathic form (the cell salt Silicea) at the same time will "teach" your body how to absorb and use the mineral silica.

### Lifestyle Support

Fungus under the nails might indicate a problem with candida throughout your whole body, which can cause fatigue and mental fuzziness in addition to physical symptoms. A good resource is **www.Needs.com**: search their articles and products for candida, and talk to their staff.

Weak and brittle nails can be one sign of overall lack of nutrients. Please follow our healthy lifestyle suggestions in Part One in addition to these localized treatments.

# NAUSEA AND VOMITING

**Quick Fix**

- Press the **acupressure point** for nausea, located on the wrist about two finger-widths up from the wrist fold, and between the two main tendons in the wrist. Keep trying until you find the tender spot.
- **Ginger** is an herb that works well for nausea, whether as a tea or fresh or powdered herb. I've used it when I'm traveling: if I'm nauseous and caught without my homeopathic kit, I'll go into a deli and buy a little nub of fresh ginger to chew on.

Or try one of these homeopathic medicines, which are likely to have other health benefits as well.

- **Nux vomica** is a good all-round choice, unless there are specific reasons to be nauseous. Nux vomica is particularly good when the person is retching with dry heaves and/or sick from too much rich fatty food.
- **Ipecac** is a great remedy for both morning sickness and nausea from fatty foods. It's a good match if the person throws up but they don't feel any better afterwards, and the tongue is clean (no "fur" or covering). Both are unusual when someone is vomiting.
- **Sepia** is likely to work if the nausea is due to morning sickness, especially if the woman is nauseous from the smell or even the thought of food (making it really hard to cook for the family), and also if the typical Sepia symptoms are present. These include a draggy-down feeling in the uterus, exhaustion, weepiness, irritability, snappishness with the loved ones, and feeling at the end of her rope. Specific symptoms during pregnancy might include lower back pain and brown skin coloration (pregnancy mask, linea nigra).

For motion sickness, see **Travel Tips.**

**Ongoing Care**

For recurring nausea, you can buy an **Acu-Band,** a wrist band with a button that presses on the point. It can work for motion sickness, morning sickness, and post-op nausea.

# NERVE PAIN AND FRAZZLED NERVES

**Quick Fix**

Hypericum works quickly for minor nerve injury, for example when you hit your finger with a hammer or damage another nerve-rich area like the lips. It can also be used for pain that shoots along the path of a nerve: dental pain which shoots from the tooth up into the jaw, or sciatica pain shooting down the sciatic nerve in the leg.

Other homeopathic medicines may work better when the nerve pain is excruciating, whereas Hypericum tends to work best for a tingling, pins-and-needles sensation. Try **Chamomilla** or **Coffea** for excruciating pain, and see pages 204–208 for directions.

**Ongoing Care**

For times when you feel "frazzled" or your "nerves are shot."

- **Coconut oil** soothes the nerves and strengthens the nervous system. It's even being used now for Alzheimer's; for a remarkable video, search YouTube for "coconut oil Alzheimer's Dr. Newport." Once lumped together with "bad" saturated fats, coconut oil is now recognized as a beneficial "medium chain fatty acid." Plus it tastes great. Pure coconut oil can be added to oatmeal or smoothies, or rubbed on the skin.

- **Kali phos.**, a tissue salt or cell salt (see page 175), is great for times when your nerves feel depleted — say when you've been studying too much and especially from using the computer too much. Or you can get these products, which include Kali phos:
  - o **Nerve Tonic by Hylands**, a blend of the five cell salts that include phosphorus, which is so important for the nervous system.
  - o **Calms Forte by Hylands,** which contains the same minerals plus a homeopathic dilution of several herbs used for hundreds of years to calm the nerves and promote sound sleep.

- Or you can get the calming herbs full strength, for example in **Traditional Medicinals' Easy Now** or **Gaia Herb's Sleep and Relax.**

## OSTEOPOROSIS AND OSTEOPENIA

**Ongoing Care**

Your bones need more than just calcium. They need a whole range of different minerals to create the lattice-like structure into which calcium is deposited, plus they need **Vitamins D3** and **K2** to help make that happen. Look for a bone-building formula such as **Jarrow Bone-Up** and pair it with **Jarrow's MK-7** (a highly bio-active form of K2). Also:

- Ipriflavone, a derivative from soy, which may prevent bone loss.
- The cell salts **Calc. phos.** (page 173) and **Silicea** (page 178). These cell salts "teach" your body to absorb calcium from your food and deposit it where it belongs in your bones.
- Or **Bio-Sil**, concentrated silica that improves calcium absorption.

**Lifestyle Support**

You know you need to take in calcium from your diet, but did you know that some foods actually make your calcium levels worse? For example, most soft drinks get their fizz from phosphates. But adding phosphorus to your diet means you need more calcium to balance it out, which may be why soft drinks contribute to osteoporosis.

Acid-causing foods (notably sugar and meat, and see Felicia Kliment's *The Acid-Alkaline Balance Diet* for the whole list) also increase your need for calcium. A high protein diet causes the body to excrete it.

The best book on nutrition and supplements for the bones is Pamela Levin's *Perfect Bones*. You can download some of her info at **www. PerfectBones.com**, including an article on tests for bone strength which are both more accurate than DEXA scans and safer (no radiation).

Weight-bearing exercise can work as well as hormone replacement therapy for strengthening bones in older women (see Dr. Miriam Nelson's *Strong Women Stay Young*). Did you know there are entire exercise programs designed to prevent and even reverse osteoporosis? The gentle exercises of **Bones for Life™** are more effective than struggling with heavy weights and they're safe enough for elderly women. Check out the demos on the GreenHealingTV channel on YouTube.

# PMS

## Quick Fix

**Aromatherapy** can be an ideal way to treat PMS since the message from the essential oils goes directly into a deep part of the brain: just one long nerve cell connects a receptor in your nose with your brain. So aromatherapy's effectiveness is practically hard-wired into your brain. It's also a relaxing modality when the oils are added to a bath or used for massage. The most medicinally active oils are not necessarily the best smelling, so you can add fragrant oils that you like.

- For swollen breasts, bloating: grapefruit, lemon, or juniper oil.
- For a PMS headache: inhale lavender, peppermint, or marjoram.
- For mood swings: clary sage, bergamot, geranium, rose. Clary sage is uplifting, bergamot helps with anxiety and mood stability, geranium helps with irritability, and rose helps with sadness and depression.
- For cramps before your period: clary sage, lavender (which also has a calming effect) and/or chamomile oils rubbed on the abdomen.

Herbalist & Alchemist's Full Moon Formula is an herbal blend for cramps with butterbur, viburnum, wild yam and chamomile.

You can also try a homeopathic remedy if you feel there's one that matches you well—and if it does, you'll probably find other things getting better as well. The remedies described under **Hormone Balancing** and **Menopause** work for PMS as well. **Sepia** works especially well for women who get weepy and irritable with PMS, **Lachesis** for women whose PMS symptoms go away the moment their period starts, and **Cimicifuga** for women who feel like they're losing their minds with PMS. **Pulsatilla** is great for the sudden moodiness of teenage girls.

Since these remedies can have such a profound overall effect, I would only try them short term (an occasional 30c remedy or 6c if you are sensitive) then discontinue if you're not getting any benefit.

## Ongoing Care

Follow the suggestions under **Hormone Balancing**.

# SCIATICA

## Quick Fix

A homeopathic remedy may be able to provide quick pain relief, but it will only be temporary because addressing the underlying condition will take time.

- Liddell's BPS ("back pain + sciatica") provides a blend of homeopathic medicines in a fast-acting oral spray. Or use a specific one:
- Hypericum for pain shooting down the leg along the path of the nerve.
- Colocynth if cramping pain makes you want to flex your leg.
- Chamomilla for excruciating pain, spasms, numbness.
- Rhus tox. or Ruta if from an injury, with stiffness from rest or damp.

## Ongoing Care

Sciatica is caused by injury to or pressure on the sciatic nerve, which goes from the spine down the leg. Treatment depends on whether the problem starts where the nerve root exits the spine, or where the nerve goes through the butt muscles. Either way, **chiropractic care** can help by stabilizing the pelvis.

Homeopathic remedies might provide lasting relief by removing factors causing compression of the nerve (no promises, but worth trying $20 worth of remedies):

- Bone spurs from the spine: **Hekla lava 6c** and **Calc. fluor. 6x** can sometimes dissolve bone spurs. (See page 173 for Calc. fluor.)
- Herniated disks: **Helodrilus 6c** (a remedy you will need to special-order) and **Calc. fluor. 6x** can strengthen disks.

In either case, take the remedies twice a day for several months.

## Preventing Recurrence

Don't put your wallet in your hip pocket and then sit on it while you drive or work, because it will impinge on the exact spot where the sciatic nerve goes through the piriformis muscle. Guys please take note of this common cause of sciatica.

Airplane seats are notoriously bad for sciatica (see page 137).

# SPLINTERS AND EMBEDDED OBJECTS

**Quick Fix**

Silica can push out anything embedded under the skin, like a splinter, a shard of glass, shrapnel, or all the little bits of gravel that get embedded in your kid's knee when he falls off his bike. One dose is often enough (a few tiny pellets dissolved in the mouth), but you can safely give a dose twice a day until the object works its way out.

The shrapnel example comes from the oldtimey homeopaths who used it in army field hospitals. Yes, in World War I and II there were homeopathic medical units in Europe who got great results using these natural medicines for wounds.

Because it can push out embedded objects, though, you have to be careful not to give it to someone with a pacemaker. It could even push out artificial joints. However, experience has shown that it will not push out IUDs or fillings in the teeth.

---

### SEA URCHIN SPINES AND SHARDS OF GLASS

A fellow homeopath gave Silica to a little girl who had fallen onto broken glass, and even after her mother picked out what she could, the little girl's hand was still filled with tiny fragments.

After the dose of Silica, at first it felt like a whole crop of little stiff hairs all over the girl's hand. Then the tiny shards of glass emerged and fell out.

I gave Silica to a friend who had stepped on a sea urchin, and the thin bony spines were embedded in her foot. A dose of Silica pushed them to the surface so that they were easy to remove.

My most dramatic experience with Silica, though, came when I gave it to a client who had a metal plate in her hand from a car accident years before when the small bones in her hand were crushed. All the tiny little titanium screws unscrewed themselves and could be felt under her skin.

Fortunately she was happy with this outcome. Her chiropractor had recommended removing the metal plate, but her insurance wouldn't cover the surgery—until the plate started to come out by itself.

# SPORTS INJURIES

**Quick Fix**

Use the following for soft tissue injury. (Sprains and strains on page 106):

∾ **Arnica** or **Traumeel** taken internally (see pages 204–208 for instructions),

∾ **Arnica, Traumeel** or **Topricin** ointment applied externally.

You can use both internal and topical treatments at the same time for faster results.

For a blow to the breast, for female athletes:

∾ **Bellis perennis,** a close cousin of Arnica, which also helps prevent and treat soreness from mammograms.

**Ongoing Care**

∾ **Sports massage** to help reduce soreness and heal the injury by increasing blood flow to the area.

∾ **Bromelain** (an enzyme from pineapples) to help repair injuries by breaking down damaged tissue, reducing swelling, and increasing blood flow.

∾ **Zinc** to repair damaged muscles, for example as L-OptiZinc, 20mg.

∾ **B vitamins** in a B-50 complex.

∾ **Vitamin D3** because a deficiency causes loss of muscle mass.

**Preventing Recurrence**

∾ **Sports massage** reduces muscle stiffness and improves muscle flexibility and range of motion in the joints, thereby reducing the likelihood of injury.

∾ **Curcumin,** the almost universally useful anti-inflammatory, also helps prevent muscle damage and muscle breakdown during workouts.

∾ **Bio-Sil,** a highly concentrated and absorbable form of silica, promotes collagen formation and strengthens joints.

∾ **Vitamin D3** helps maintain muscle mass.

## SPRAINS AND STRAINS

### Quick Fix

∾ **Topricin, Traumeel** or **Castro's Joint Cream** (see **Arthritis**). Then find the best-matching homeopathic remedy for your type of pain:

∾ **Rhus tox.**, the most common remedy for sprains, strains and joint pains, is called the "rusty gate remedy." People who need it feel stiff and need to limber up or apply heat (a hot bath or heating pad). They typically wake up feeling stiff and have to do stretching exercises to get going.

∾ **Ruta grav.** is similar to Rhus tox. It has a special affinity for the knee joint and it's the best remedy if your knee "pops" or gives out from underneath you, often without pain, perhaps while you are going downstairs. It can also help with plantar fasciitis (which causes pain in the heel and sole of the foot).

∾ **Bryonia** has the opposite quality so it's easy to tell them apart. People who need Bryonia feel more pain from the slightest movement. So they do what we call "guarding"—they try to hold the body part absolutely still to avoid more pain. They are often irritable from the pain and want to be left alone—the "grouchy bear in the cave."

### Ongoing Care

If the joint pain is recent, say from a sprained ankle, you can relieve the pain and speed up the healing with natural remedies. If the joint pain is chronic, say from arthritis or fibromyalgia, you can get temporary relief to tide you over while seeking professional help from a naturopath or homeopath.

In other words, don't expect to cure longstanding joint problems with these home remedies, but they are safe to try and may provide you with good short-term relief.

Nutritional support for injured joints includes **essential fatty acids** and **glucosamine/chondroitin** (see **Arthritis**). You may need **chiropractic care** to fix your biomechanics if you keep injuring yourself.

# STINGS, HIVES, AND ITCHY SKIN

## Quick Fix

- **Seven Cream** is an amazing skin cream for lots of itchy and/or dry skin conditions, including poison ivy, insect bites, even eczema and psoriasis. My clients have reported great results using it for all of these conditions. It's not expected to *cure* longterm conditions, but it can give you great *relief* while you're seeking professional help from a holistic health care professional.
- **Aloe vera gel** soothes many skin conditions. Keep it in the refrigerator for an extra cooling effect.
- **An oatmeal bath** relieves itching: powder a cup of rolled oats in the blender and pour into a hot bath. Oats contain a natural itch-reliever.
- **Apis** is the most likely homeopathic remedy to work for red, swollen bumps that may feel warm to the touch and burning and/or itchy to the person—in other words, things that look like a bee sting but might be hives. Apis can work whether it's an insect bite or an allergic reaction because the symptoms are more important than the diagnosis in using homeopathic medicines. (See directions on pages 204–208.) It can even stave off anaphylactic shock in an emergency when there's no epi pen available.
- **Histaminum** is like a generic anti-histamine.
- For specific triggers: try **Arsenicum** for hives from strawberries, **Sepia** for hives during pregnancy or other hormonal events, **Urtica** for hives from shellfish, **Pulsatilla** if from pork or rich, fatty foods.
- As for insect bites, **Apis** works best if the area is warm, whereas **Ledum** is more likely to work if it's cool to the touch; Apis if the swelling is pink or reddish, Ledum if it's purplish.

## Ongoing Care

**Nettles** have a great anti-histamine effect. You want to get good quality freeze-dried nettles such as **Eclectic Institute's**. **Vitamin C** and **quercetin** can reduce allergic reactions.

## Lifestyle Support

Speaking of psoriasis and eczema, it's beyond the scope of this book to cover treating them, but I'll give you some hints to get you started.

Psoriasis is related to toxins building up in the body. When the primary routes of elimination (liver, kidneys and colon) get backed up, the body starts to use the skin as an alternate route. Dr. John Pagano's *Healing Psoriasis: The Natural Alternative* is based on this approach, and I know people for whom it has worked. They also feel healthier overall and have more energy from the cleansing and healthy diet he recommends. **Gaia Herb's Liver Support** and **Terry Naturally Curamed Curcumin** will get your cleanse off to a great start and possibly heal minor cases of psoriasis.

I know people whose psoriasis has totally cleared up just from homeopathy, some of whom had previously benefited from the Pagano diet but who could not stick to it. Eczema can also be relieved with a nutritional or homeopathic approach from a holistic professional.

### "I COULD HAVE BOUGHT A HOUSE"

A graphic designer in her late thirties came to see me for psoriasis, for which she had already tried just about everything under the sun — conventional medications, ultraviolet light therapy, and a long list of alternative treatments. She had had psoriasis for nearly 30 years, and she figured she had spent about $200,000 on it. "I could have bought a house!" as she put it.

Over the next year and a half her psoriasis gradually went away until only one spot was left, the spot over her left eyebrow where it had begun when she was 11. This was a beautiful example of how homeopathy can "put your health history on rewind" and go back to the beginning, to the roots, of a health condition.

## SURGERY: PRE-OP AND POST-OP

**Quick Fix**

∾ **Arnica** for bruising, soreness, and swelling. It's especially good for preventing bruising after plastic surgery, and apparently a lot of plastic surgeons are using it now.

∾ **Calendula** to heal the incision, prevent infection and scarring, and reduce pain.

∾ **Phosphorus** to help you come out of the anesthesia and to prevent excessive bleeding afterwards. (You may or may not need Phosphorus depending on the type of surgery and your own experience with coming out of anesthesia.)

Directions. one dose of each beforehand (for complete instructions see page 211). Afterwards focus on the one you need most. Phosphorus first, if at all, then **Arnica** as long as there is bruising, soreness and swelling—maybe a few days.

Give **Calendula** orally, and also make a water solution to soak the dressing with, until the surgical incision is completely healed.

If you want to be sure to prevent scarring, use Miranda Castro's **Scar Cream**, available online. Castro tells me that her local plastic surgeon buys it by the case because he gets such good results with it.

If you're having laser surgery on your eyes, use Aconite before and after instead of Arnica. You can find more on eye surgery in Dr. Edward Kondrot's *Healing the Eye the Natural Way* and *Ten Essentials for Improving Your Eyesight,* **www.HealingTheEye.com**.

**Ongoing care**

Before you go in for surgery, get *Prepare for Surgery, Heal Faster* by Peggy Huddleston. The book and CD provide relaxation exercises that will help you be less anxious beforehand and also have less pain and recover more quickly afterwards. You will even bleed less during surgery, as documented by hundreds of studies done on thousands of patients using this method. Many hospitals now have nurses trained to teach it to patients.

# TEETHING

## Quick Fix

Hyland's Teething Tablets or Teething Gel are old favorites, and they were among the most popular products in my health food store.

They are a combination of several possible remedies for teething, which increases the chances that at least one of them will work. Sometimes, though, the *single, specific* homeopathic remedy works better than a blend:

- **Chamomilla** for pain so intense the child is in a raging fit, demanding things then throwing them on the floor.
- **Belladonna** is another teething remedy with dramatic symptoms: sudden onset, high fever, red face, possibly dilated pupils, possibly angry and biting.
- **Calc. carb.** if the teething doesn't seem to hurt so much and especially if the child matches the Calc. carb. type. They tend to have a calm, even lethargic temperament and lots of baby fat. They tend to do everything late—walking, talking, teething—because they like to take their own sweet time.

## Ongoing Care

The cell salt **Calc. phos.** (see page 173) can make the teething process easier by strengthening the teeth and helping them erupt through the gums faster.

### INSTANT RELIEF FOR A TEETHING BABY

I've heard many stories from the parents of my little clients about how much their children love taking homeopathic medicines. It's not unusual for a four- or five-year-old to have mastered the names of the medicines she usually needs and to ask for one by name when she feels sick. (These Latin names! Can you imagine?)

It's also not unusual for a toddler to toddle over to the cupboard where the medicines are stored and pat the cupboard door to indicate he wants a remedy.

Here's my favorite story, though. The mother of a 10-month-old infant was already using Hyland's Teething Tablets when she brought her baby to see me for another issue. She mentioned that the baby seemed to have learned the sound of the pellets rattling in the tube. He would be crying with teething pain, then hear the rattle of the pellets as she got out the tube.

Instantly cries would turn into a big smile as the baby kicked and waved with glee knowing that relief was on the way. This was before she even gave him a dose!

---

### HUGS INSTEAD OF EAR TUBES

*This story comes from Donna Thompson, my colleague who contributed the Flower Essence section of this book.*

My nephew had so many ear infections, he was scheduled for surgery to put tubes in his ears. This was when I was studying homeopathy, and I wanted to treat *everybody.* But his mother was afraid to give him a remedy because she was very fearful of any medication and especially of something her doctor was not familiar with. Of course there isn't actually anything *in it,* but she was being careful about something she didn't understand.

Finally she let me give him one dose of Chamomilla. When he went for his pre-op visit, the doctor was amazed—his ears were totally clear. He never had another ear infection and he never needed the surgery.

What's more, he had previously been tested as having hearing loss from the fluid in his ears. After this one dose of Chamomilla, his hearing came back 100%.

Here's the best part, though. Before the remedy, he would never hug people, especially someone he didn't see much. A few months after the remedy, at a Christmastime family get together, he came up and gave me a hug and a smile. Everyone stopped talking and watched because it was so surprising to see him do this.

His mom confirmed that he had become more affectionate with her too. Before, he was angry all the time, demanding and reactive, always acting out with her. After the remedy he calmed down and told her that he loved her.

# THUMBSUCKING

## Quick Fix

**Pulsatilla** covers thumbsucking when it's part of a larger picture: a child who wants to remain babyish and has the typical Pulsatilla personality (clingy, attached to mom, cuddly and affectionate, generally sweet and mild tempered but can also be whiny and manipulative and suddenly teary). Children may tend to be like this from birth, especially if they experienced abandonment as a newborn (for example from a Caesarian or from being dropped off at daycare too soon).

Or they may develop regressive tendencies when a new baby sister or brother starts getting all the attention, and somewhere in their little brain they figure out that acting like a baby might get them back in the limelight again. For these kids, thumbsucking might be part of a pattern that includes forgetting their potty training, wanting to drink from a bottle again, and wanting to sleep in mommy and daddy's bed again. Not to mention clinging like a little barnacle to mom's leg when dropped off at daycare.

For a child like this, Pulsatilla is not just about fixing the thumbsucking. It's about relieving the child's feeling of abandonment, whether from birth, or from losing their special spot in their parents' affection when a new baby appears.

## Ongoing Support

There might be a totally different reason, though, with a different fix. Thumbsucking stimulates the point in the roof of the mouth between the hard and soft palate. Above that point is the hypothalamus, which releases endorphins, the body's natural pain-relievers and stress-reducers. Sometimes the system doesn't work, though, and the child has found that the palate needs to be rubbed to release those innate stress relievers. Take your child to a **craniosacral therapist**, or to a **non-force chiropractor for a "sphenobasilar adjustment."** Bring this book along, just in case they haven't heard of this connection (which I learned about from my very smart craniosacral and chiropractic colleagues).

# TOOTH PROBLEMS

## Quick Fix for Tooth Pain

- **Clove oil** applied directly to the tooth is a traditional remedy for toothaches (may not be safe for teething babies, though).
- **Chamomilla,** the top homeopathic remedy for excruciating pain during teething, works for adults too, especially if they're cranky.
- **Coffea** is a backup plan for these excruciating toothaches, more for people who tend to be nervous and hypersensitive and sleepless.
- **Mercurius** is a great remedy for any problem in the mouth with typical symptoms of excessive salivation, mouth sores, bleeding gums, bad breath, scalloped edges of the tongue, and a possible recent exposure to mercury such as from a filling being replaced.

## Avoiding a Root Canal

If you have a toothache but the dentist can't find any signs of infection, he may say, "There's nothing wrong, but if it still hurts, we can do a root canal." If you're like most people and dread getting a root canal more than anything, even public speaking, this tip is for you.

A toothache without infection may indicate a jammed tooth. For example, you just got a permanent crown put on, and they jammed the new tooth down hard onto your old tooth. Or maybe there was a blow or an injury. If so, you may have a tooth that's jammed like a peg in a hole. Here's a tip from my chiropractic colleagues.

You pull the tooth away from the socket (it will only move a tiny bit) and wiggle it in all directions: back and forth, to and fro. You'll need to keep doing it over several weeks, even months. But you may be able to loosen the tooth enough to stop the pain and save the tooth.

But what if you really do need a root canal? Some of my clients have reported avoiding one with an herbal combination called **Padma,** available online. Don't go AWOL from your dentist while trying to avoid a root canal on your own, though. Find out from your dentist how urgent the situation is. Make sure your dentist is monitoring the situation.

## Tooth Infections

In an emergency, if you can't get to dental care and have an infected tooth, use the homeopathic infection series: **Belladonna** for the first stage (throbbing pain, maybe swollen and warm), **Hepar sulph.** for the second stage (you're irritable and extremely sensitive to anything touching the area) and then when it's come to a head, **Silica** to push out the pus. You can get them in any health food store; follow directions on pages 204-208 and put them in water to speed up the process.

## Tooth Extractions

Follow the directions for **Surgery: Pre-Op and Post-Op.** I have recommended **Arnica, Calendula,** and **Phosphorus** to many friends and clients undergoing tooth extractions. They have needed fewer pain-killers afterwards, some needed none at all—and their mouths tended to heal quickly. (See directions on page 211.) **Ruta grav.** or **clove oil** will help if you get a condition called "dry socket" after the extraction.

## Gum Disease

Did you ever wonder what people did before toothbrushes and dentists? In the Middle East, they used a *miswak* or **"chewing stick."** These sticks are now available online and are pleasant to rub on your teeth and gums. Apparently lots of studies have documented that they work better than a toothbrush for reducing plaque and bacteria in the mouth and for preventing gum disease.

## Braces Tightened

If your child's teeth, jaw, or even head hurts after her braces are tightened, try **Ruta grav.** This natural medicine targets the connective tissue surrounding bones and teeth. Tightening braces stresses the whole system: teeth, jaw, and even the bones of the skull. That's why some kids get headaches after their braces are tightened.

Ruta grav. can help to some extent, although this is basically a structural problem best treated by a chiropractor or craniosacral therapist. I recommend bringing your child for a **craniosacral or chiropractic adjustment** if she has a headache after her braces are tightened.

# TRAVEL TIPS

## Quick Fixes

You might want to take the following medicines with you, along with the directions on pages 204–208.

- ∾ **Arsenicum** for traveler's diarrhea (more on this, page 184).
- ∾ **Nux vomica** for upset stomachs from unfamiliar food.
- ∾ **Arnica – Calendula – Phosphorus**, the injury trio.
- ∾ **Carbo veg.** if you are going to a higher altitude where you may have difficulty breathing, because this medicine helps your body absorb oxygen more effectively.
- ∾ **Jet Zone** or **No Jet Lag**, available in any health food store and many drug stores for jet lag.
- ∾ **Apis** if your feet swell up on the plane so you can't get your shoes back on.
- ∾ **Causticum** if you get sick on the plane with hoarseness and a dry cough. Causticum is a great remedy for getting sick from a cold dry wind — like the blower right above your head on the plane.
- ∾ **Cocculus** is good for motion sickness, especially when associated with a forward-backward lurching, as on a bus. It's also great for jet lag, so you don't need a separate jet lag remedy if you're getting Cocculus for motion sickness. Take a dose before takeoff, another one on landing, and additional doses on an "as needed" basis for shifting your internal time clock.
- ∾ **Tabacum** or **Petroleum** are more likely to work for motion sickness from side-to-side pitching as on a boat. It's easy to remember the difference: Tabacum is used for people who feel better breathing in fresh air (imagine going up on deck for a smoke), while Petroleum is for people who want to stay inside or below decks (imagine being down by the boat engine and getting sick from the fumes). Tabacum is also good for what's called "deathly nausea" when the person looks almost green, they are so sick. (Remember your first cig? did you throw up?)

∾ Liddell's homeopathic motion sickness spray combines Cocculus, Tabacum, Petroleum and several other remedies in an oral spray which works quickly.

**Airplane seats** are notoriously bad for sciatica and lower back pain. Bring along a wedge pillow, or roll up a sweater and place it in the small of your back to keep your lower back arched. Also my chiropractic colleagues recommend not eating sugar before or during a flight. They say that sugar destabilizes the sacrum, which creates a bad combination with that cramped airplane seat.

**Ears popping:** Check the **Ear Problems** section, page 86, for what to do if your ears are blocked before you take off.

**Outback medicine:** If you will be doing extensive traveling, especially to a Third World country or outback where you may not have access to good medical care, study Colin Lessel's *World Traveler's Manual of Homeopathy* ahead of time. It covers much more than homeopathy. It will tell you what diseases you may encounter for each country plus supplies to bring for emergency medical care.

# TUMMY TROUBLES AND FOOD POISONING

## Quick Fix

- Herbal remedies for indigestion include **chewable peppermint enzymes, ginger,** and digestive bitters such as **Underberg Bitters.**
- **Nux vomica** is the first homeopathic to try for most stomach problems, except in one of the following scenarios:
- If food poisoning is involved, think first of **Arsenicum.** People who need Arsenicum are likely to be anxious and restless and to have burning pains. People who need Nux vomica, on the other hand, are likely to be irritable with spasmodic cramping.
- **Pulsatilla** for a child who fits the Pulsatilla profile (clingy, cuddly, affectionate, whiny) who might be using her tummy upset as an excuse for special attention. She may honestly feel sick, but when mom's special attention is her best medicine, Pulsatilla can speed up the cure.

Remember that throwing up can be the body's way to protect itself against, say, spoiled food. If you give a remedy and the person throws up right away, maybe the remedy gave the body extra strength to do what it needed to do anyway.

## Ongoing Care

If you are traveling to a country where food poisoning is likely to be a problem, here's what you can do to protect yourself:

- Take a preventive dose of **Arsenicum 30c** on each day that you're likely to be exposed to bad food or water. (If you are very sensitive to homeopathy, use a lower dose, **Arsenicum 6c.**)
- Or take along a bottle of **echinacea extract** and put a dropperful into each glass of water you drink, for its protective effects.
- In any case, take a daily dose of a good strong **probiotic.**
- Be careful with bottled water, which in Third World countries may just be tap water. Ice cubes are probably not made with pure water.
- Avoid eating food from street vendors and stick to tourist hotels.

# URINARY INCONTINENCE

## Quick Fix

**Causticum** for "stress incontinence" in older adults. (This means leaking a bit of urine when you sneeze or cough or laugh. Don't laugh, it's really common in older women.)

It has worked almost across the board for my clients, however it's *especially* likely to work when the person has the typical Causticum emotional symptoms: anxiety about the welfare of family members and/or a sense of injustice and of fighting for the underdog.

Another good option: **Enur-Aid by Hylands** is a combination homeopathic that includes half a dozen medicines likely to help with urinary incontinence.

## Ongoing Care

**Equisetum** (horsetail) tincture strengthens the muscles of the bladder and helps improve control. Take a dropperful twice a day in water or juice.

## Lifestyle Support

If natural medicines don't work, **chiropractic** adjustments can help with bowel and bladder problems in older adults, especially if there has been an injury to the lower back (where the nerves come out that go to the bowel and bladder). Or there may be an injury to the pubic bones, typically from falling onto the crotch (for example from falling onto the crossbar of a bike). My colleagues at Lydian Chiropractic have cured many a case of incontinence by adjusting dislodged pubic bones.

If an older man loses bladder control after prostate surgery, presumably the nerves to that area were damaged during the surgery. In that case it will be harder, maybe impossible to bring back bladder control, but still worth a try.

# URINARY TRACT INFECTIONS

## Quick Fix

~ **Cantharis** is the most widely used natural medicine for UTIs. It covers the typical symptoms of frequency and urgency, with a cutting or burning pain, and the urine may even feel hot as it comes out—typically drop by drop. It may have a little blood in it. The pain may be excruciating. Don't panic yet—try Cantharis, but if your natural remedies don't work and you have a substantial amount of blood, go see your doctor.

~ **Apis** is another likely candidate, especially if there is edema (swelling) anywhere in the body (fingers, ankles) or a sore, swollen abdomen painful to the touch.

~ **Sarsaparilla** is a medicine you'll need to special-order to have on hand, if you typically get UTIs which are really painful at the *end* of urination.

~ **Sepia** will match best if you have typical Sepia symptoms (exhausted, overworked, feeling like you have not a minute to yourself, you need a vacation, you are draggy and even your bladder and uterus feel like they are sliding down). Especially likely for UTIs during pregnancy or postpartum.

~ **Staphysagria** works best for what used to be called "honeymoon cystitis" (UTIs after lots of sex, but of course many people don't wait for their honeymoon anymore). The urine may feel like it's rolling down drop by drop, and/or you may always feel like there's more in there that won't come out. Sensitive people, or anyone with a history of abuse or of suppressed anger, should use Staphysagria in a low potency (strength) such as 6c because a higher potency (30c) may bring out suppressed memories or anger.

If one of the above homeopathic medicines matches your symptoms well, your UTI should be on its way to clearing up after a couple of days. See pages 204-208 for directions on taking them.

~ If you like herbal teas, try **corn silk tea.** You can get it in a health food store, or you make your own by storing the silk from ears of corn in the freezer, then boiling a handful when you have signs of a UTI. It can work quickly like the medicines above.

## Ongoing Care

~ **Cranberry juice** helps treat and prevent urinary tract infections because it contains a plant nutrient that makes the infection slide right on out instead of sticking to the walls of your urinary tract. It's really sour, though. Sugar-sweetened commercial cranberry juice is not a great idea because sugar weakens your immune system. Some people can handle unsweetened cranberry juice from the health food store. Mixing it with a sweet juice like organic apple juice can make it go down easier.

~ There's a better way, though: concentrated cranberry capsules, which may contain the equivalent of a gallon of cranberry juice. **Solaray Cran-Actin** is a good brand.

~ Or cranberry plus traditional herbs for the urinary tract (parsley, bearberry, goldenseal, golden rod) in **Vibrant Health UT-Vibrance.**

~ Several thousand extra units of **Vitamin C** will also help.

Be on the lookout for a kidney infection (page 48) which is a serious condition requiring medical care. If your symptoms do not clear up and you develop kidney pain, see a doctor immediately.

## Preventing Recurrence

If you get frequent urinary tract infections, consider the following:

~ Take **cranberry caps** on a regular basis.

~ Use a high potency **probiotic** (each capsule has *billions,* not just millions, of organisms) such as Jarro-Dophilus or MegaFood's MegaFlora.

~ Wipe front to back (women), wear cotton underwear.

~ Be sure to drink plenty of water to keep your bladder flushed out.

~ Eat foods that will create a more alkaline urine (see Felicia Kliment's *The Acid-Alkaline Balance Diet*).

## THE CASE OF THE MYSTERIOUS
## URINARY TRACT INFECTIONS

A young woman came to see me for recurring urinary tract infections. Or at least that was the diagnosis from her doctor. She had some of the typical symptoms of urinary tract infections, including frequency and urgency. (If you've ever had one, you'll recognize those symptoms: you feel like you really, really have to pee right away, you run to the bathroom, nothing much comes out, and five minutes later you have to pee again.)

However, the drugs for urinary tract infections weren't working. As a homeopath, I listened carefully to her symptoms and also considered the larger picture, what we call the Never Well Since. The symptoms started after she came to Cambridge from Tibet to study at a distinguished university. There was a lot of grief in her story, including leaving behind her family, her friends and her homeland, plus the losses her family suffered as a result of the Chinese occupation of Tibet.

It was difficult to get specific symptoms from her because she did not speak English well and was clearly shy about talking about that area of her body. However, her story seemed to indicate the homeopathic medicine Causticum, which we use for "repetitive grief" (multiple experiences of grief and loss) and also for injustice situations, as the Tibetans have certainly experienced.

The only problem was that it didn't work. Even though I gave it to her in ever-stronger doses, and had her repeat it more often, it didn't seem to make a dent in her symptoms.

So I went back over my case notes again. I had overlooked another possible Never Well Since. The symptoms also started after she injured her back moving a filing cabinet at her work-study job.

I asked the chiropractor in my office to show me where the nerves came out of the spine that would control the bladder. Bingo! Right where the young woman had injured her back.

I referred her to the chiropractor and after just a few adjustments, the Tibetan student was free of her "urinary tract infections"—and also of the back pain which she had neglected to mention.

# VARICOSE VEINS

## Quick Fix

**Witch hazel extract** (it's an old herbal remedy and drugstores still have it). Better yet, get a stronger version of the same thing from a health food store: **Hamamelis** (witch hazel) tincture, which you'll need to dilute in a little water if it stings. Either way, rub the liquid right onto the varicose veins to tighten them up.

## Ongoing Care

Varicose veins occur when the veins in the leg sag. You can continue the witch hazel or Hamamelis (it's safe) and add **Calc. fluor. 6x,** the cell salt that strengthens elastic tissue like the walls of the veins. (See page 179 for instructions.)

For extra help, try the herbal/homeopathic Natural Treatment Protocol for Spider and Varicose Veins, which includes both a topical application and oral doses, from Homeopathic Educational Services, **www.Homeopathic.com.**

## Lifestyle Support

It helps to elevate your legs as much as possible: for example, prop up the foot of your bed with bricks or boards. My father the vascular surgeon used to say, "Keep your toes higher than your nose." Also get in the habit of elevating your legs while talking on the phone or watching TV.

If you have to work on your feet all day, you may need **compression stockings** because they help to keep the blood flowing back up to your heart instead of pooling in the veins of your legs. **Smart Wool** is the best brand because wool breathes and it's antifungal and antimicrobial (unlike the old synthetic stockings). Plus they feel luscious on your ankles and legs (**www.SmartWool.com**).

**Massage sandals** (available online) may be even more helpful because the little rubber prongies on the sole stimulate the reflexology points on the feet, which feels like it helps get the circulation going back up towards the heart.

## VISION PROBLEMS

### Quick Fix

**New glasses,** but maybe not in the "direction" you were expecting. Most people get stronger and stronger glasses, which makes their vision weaker and weaker as they get more and more dependent on their glasses. Instead, you can strengthen your eye muscles and in many cases you can overcome the need for glasses altogether.

To do this, you need to find a behavioral optometrist, in other words an optometrist trained in giving you a personalized exercise routine for your eyes. You can find a brief explanation of the method and a referral list at **www.VisionTherapy.org.** If you can't find a behavioral optometrist nearby, you can try the exercises in *Greater Vision* by Grossman and McCabe.

### Ongoing Care

Strengthen your eyes with a "vision walk": walk unimpeded, so your arms can swing freely (no packages, no briefcase, no leash). Look at something in the distance—a tree, a phone pole—and as you walk, keep your head and your eyes pointed straight ahead, while you keep the object in the corner of your eye. As you come alongside the object, you will find that you can keep "looking" straight ahead, but you will still "see" the object beside you with your peripheral vision.

Developing peripheral vision also helps the brain to hold the "big picture" instead of becoming overfocused on details.

The eyes are extremely demanding of nutrients: good sources include **Gaia Herb's Vision Enhancement** and **Solgar Bilberry-Ginkgo-Eyebright Complex.**

Stress has a direct effect on the eye (because the stress hormone adrenaline targets the eye muscles). Stress-related vision problems may be treated with **homeopathy.** If a child has one eye that turns in or out, and the child has been through an extreme emotional trauma, homeopathy may fix the eye problem by relieving the underlying emotional stress. This requires professional homeopathic care.

# WARTS AND SKIN TAGS

**Quick Fix**

I've combined these two conditions because they may respond to the same homeopathic medicine, Thuja. I've had clients on Thuja for a chronic complaint who report at the followup, "And by the way, all my warts fell off at the same time." Same with skin tags (little benign growths on your skin).

You can get Thuja ointment at your local health food store (or special-order it) and apply it directly to your warts or skin tags. Or get Thuja in pellet form, dissolve 2 pellets in a little water, and apply it externally. You might soak the gauze of a bandage with the Thuja water and then bandage your warts.

Thuja is the most common homeopathic medicine for warts, but there are others, depending on the specific location. They are not available in ointment form, however you can easily make a water dilution and apply them externally.

- **Antimonium crud.** is for plantar warts (on the soles of the feet) and warts on the hands, including around or under the nails. They tend to be hard and horny (no snickering! this means the skin is thick and dry, like scar tissue).

- **Causticum** can also work for warts on the hands, especially next to the nails; also warts on the face, even on the nose. These warts might be more likely to bleed or ooze.

- **Nitric acid** covers warts on the hands and face, plus on the genitals (although Thuja is a champ when it comes to anything in the genital area). Nitric acid-type warts are likely to be painful, cracked, bleeding, and/or itchy compared to the more benign warts that respond to Thuja.

These last three can be taken internally in a 30c potency, but Thuja will work better applied to the specific spot where it is needed.

## Ongoing Care

Apparently warts don't like sulphur, which you can take in the form of MSM or l-cysteine (500 mg, twice a day). Since warts are caused by viruses, you could take extra zinc and selenium (remember that selenium is "birth control for viruses").

## Preventing Recurrence

If your body has an ongoing tendency to produce warts or skin tags, this is part of a larger health pattern which homeopathy is especially well-designed to treat. In the process you are likely to find an improvement in your overall health and energy level.

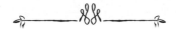

## Part Three

# STOCKING YOUR NATURAL MEDICINE CABINET

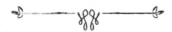

In Part Three, you'll learn the best products to put in your natural medicine cabinet. I've tried to make it simple so that you feel empowered to plunge in and start.
I recommend getting the products on the next page so you have them on hand when emergencies come up.

Speaking of simple, the easiest way to get familiar with homeopathic remedies is with the combination remedies for specific conditions. They're easy to spot because they usually have clever names based on their usage, and they are almost foolproof, as you'll see from my description.

Then I'll give you a more complete description of the items on the "short list" plus a few more favorite herbs and homeopathics.

Then there's a special section on flower essences, which appeared earlier in the Emotional First Aid section, and which deserve more coverage because they are so useful for a wide range of emotional states.

Another special section explains cell salts, which many people like to begin experimenting with because they are so safe (it's impossible to take too much of them) and manageable (only 12 of them).

# STARTING YOUR NATURAL MEDICINE CABINET: THE SHORT LIST

To keep it simple, here's what I recommend keeping on hand when you're just starting with natural healing:

- ~ Aloe vera gel
- ~ Calendula cream
- ~ Elderberry syrup
- ~ Insure Herbal
- ~ Rescue Remedy
- ~ Topricin or Traumeel ointment
- ~ Calms Forte
- ~ Ferrum phos. 6x cell salt
- ~ Arnica
- ~ Arsenicum
- ~ Gelsemium
- ~ Hypericum
- ~ Ignatia
- ~ Kali bic.
- ~ Nux vomica
- ~ Phosphorus

And for nutritional support:

- ~ A good multivitamin
- ~ Fish oil or plant-based essential fatty acids
- ~ Calcium/magnesium
- ~ Vitamin C
- ~ Vitamin D3
- ~ Vitamin E
- ~ A probiotic
- ~ A green food powder

These products are all available in health food stores. Get the homeopathic remedies (Arnica through Phosphorus) in a 30c potency or strength, which is ideal for most people.

# COMBINATION REMEDIES:
# QUICK AND EASY

Combination remedies are the quickest way to get started with homeo-pathic medicines, which in turn are the quickest way to get results with natural healing. These blends include the top medicines for a condition, with handy names that give you a big clue as to what they are for, like Pollinosan for pollen allergies or Cyclease for menstrual cramps. Your health food store, and maybe even your pharmacy, will have a whole section of them. Here are some of my favorites:

- **Calms Forte** for insomnia and for feeling calmer during the day
- **Teething Tabs** and **Teething Gel** by Hylands, which are universal mothers' favorites
- **Alpha CF:** CF stands for Colds and Flu, and this was a top favorite in my health food store
- **Jet Zone** or No Jet Lag
- **Topricin** or **Traumeel** for sports injuries, sprains and strains, pulled muscles, sore muscles

Traumeel is made by Heel, a German company that does excellent research on its products (and its name comes from "trauma" plus "Heel"). Their homeopathic combinations often work as well as, or even better than, the conventional medicine for the same condition. For example:

- **Vertigoheel** for vertigo

- ∾ **Sinusin** nasal spray for nasal congestion and sinusitis
- ∾ **Zeel** for joint stiffness and arthritic pain
- ∾ **Cerecomp** for mental fatigue and lack of concentration
- ∾ **Exhaustion** for stress, insomnia and overexertion as well as fatigue.

Another of my favorite brands is NatraBio, which makes the highly effective bioAllers blends described in the Allergy section. Some of their other popular products in my health food store were **Smoking Cessation** and **Caffeine Withdrawal**, to relieve the withdrawal symptoms.

Here's the deal. These combination products work.

Well, they work if they match your condition, because homeopathic medicines have to match specific symptoms. Let's take coughs, for example. A homeopathic medicine can stop a cough dead in its tracks if it matches your symptoms perfectly. Do you have a dry cough or a rattly cough? Does it rattle in the middle of your chest or at the base of your lungs? Are you coughing up green yucky stuff or white slimy stuff? Do you cough when you talk, or breathe in cold air, or lie down on your back? Are you tired of answering questions yet?

Depending on your answer to these and many other questions, you might need any one of maybe 50 different cough remedies. Each company making a cough formula picks the top 5 or 7 remedies, in their view. If your specific cough remedy is in the formula, you're in luck, and it will probably work fabulously for you. If not, maybe it contains a remedy with *similar* symptoms to your cough — if so, the blend may take the edge off your cough but not totally stop it. Or maybe the blend doesn't work for you because none of the remedies match or it's not strong enough (or in homeo-speak, it's not in a high enough potency).

So if you buy one of these blends and it doesn't work, please don't say that homeopathy doesn't work. It just means that that particular blend didn't have the medicine you needed, in the strength you needed. No harm — save it for a friend or family member. It may work for them. And don't worry about the expiration date, which is just a legal technicality with homeopathic medicines.

Try another blend by a different company. Get out your magnifying glass and read the ingredients in the fine print on the back. Some companies even tell you the specific symptom for each ingredient. You'll notice that each brand has a different ingredient list because they have a different idea as to which medicines will work the best. With blends for pollen allergies, for example, pollens vary by geographical area, season, and weather. Ask the staff at your local health food store which blend seems to be working best for people in your area.

On the whole, though, this "combination approach" is a great way to get started. You'll feel empowered when it works and you'll get comfortable with homeopathy. The blends are inexpensive, typically $8 to $15, so you might want to pick up several of them while you're in the store and experiment when you get home. Once you find the one that works for you, you have a friend for life.

So why wouldn't you just stick with this approach, buying a cleverly-labeled concoction for each of your health problems? Here's why:

- Taking more than one homeopathic medicine at a time "blurs the information" from the one your body needs.
- Working with single medicines rather than combinations, you may well find a medicine that helps you across the board, with different health conditions, because many homeopathic medicines affect more than one body part.
- The combinations use low (weak) potencies and they may not be strong enough for you.
- You may need an unusual medicine which is not found in any combination.

Let me explain.

Homeopathic medicines work because of the information they give your body, rather than conveying medicinal "stuff" the way a drug or an herb or vitamin would. They all contain the same simple ingredients — sugar, water, maybe a little alcohol. No drugs in there! What's in there is *information*, sort of like the information stored on a computer chip. More about this in **How Do the Remedies Work?**, page 212.

When you're sick, your body's healing energy has been thrown off by something, perhaps a cold wind, or food poisoning, or upsetting news. Your body's healing energy creates symptoms while struggling to get back in balance. Along comes the homeopathic medicine. It's like the blueprint, the template for what it's like to be healthy. Your body knows how to be healthy, it just needs to be reminded. It wants to get the message, the information, from the homeopathic medicine.

But what if there are half a dozen messages coming through at the same time? It's like getting more than one station on the radio. It's hard to hear the one you want. A single homeopathic medicine gives your body's healing energy the information it needs *more* effectively than a blend. Note that this is very different from herbal medicine. Herbs work better in blends because each plant contains ingredients that add to the effects of the others.

There's a way to get around this problem of the different medicines competing with each other to get their message across. That's by "turning down the volume" on each one, providing it in a low potency (low dosage, in drug terms). But then it might not be strong enough to work for you.

Get out your magnifying glass again and look at the ingredients on the back. Each of the long Latin names is followed by a number, typically 3 or 6. Then go to the section of the store with single homeopathic medicines. Look at the numbers on their labels. Probably 30, right? That's a lot stronger than 3 or 6.

Occasionally you will find combinations with high numbers like 200. Personally, I don't think it's wise to take these high-potency remedies multiple times a day as the label may recommend. They are just too strong, at least for some people. An occasional one-time dose is fine, but combinations are usually taken several times a day for a week or more. The low potencies are better for frequent usage. (Exception: some people are strong as an ox and just don't feel anything unless they use high potencies. You will learn this by experience.)

So please, start off with the combinations with the intention that you will "graduate" into the wonderful world of single homeopathic medicines. They are like beautiful tuning forks or bells which can resonate through your whole being and bring you back to health, harmony, and balance. The most widely used single remedies are described in the last chapter in this section.

# A HANDFUL OF HEALING HERBS

There are many ways to enjoy the healing benefits of medicinal herbs. They have traditionally been used together in blends because each one has a different array of active ingredients which support each other synergistically. So the easiest way to use them if you're a busy person is to find a combination designed for your health issue, made by a company you trust.

I highly recommend Gaia Herbs because I know with what care they are made. The plants are grown in a pristine environment (a remote valley in North Carolina, watered by pure streams flowing off the mountaintop), carefully tended and harvested, and with their active ingredients tested by a team of research scientists.

This is important because the amount of medicinal ingredients in an herb can vary widely depending on many conditions, including the quality of the soil, the weather during the growing season, the species of the plant, the part of the plant used, and when the plant was harvested (time of year, time of day, even the phase of the moon). So you want to trust your herb grower to create the best possible conditions for the most effective herbs.

A simple way to get started with herbs is with combinations like **Gaia Herb's Migra-profen** (headaches and body aches and pains), **Sound Sleep, Reflux Relief, Gas & Bloating,** and **Natural Laxative.** Your health food store will have lots of herbal formulas for various ills.

Let's say you want to handle the plants directly, though, rather than getting the herbs already encapsulated. There's something very healing about connecting with nature by starting with a living plant and creating your own medicinals. You can learn to make your own tinctures and teas, your ointments and salves, depending on your favorite tastes and fragrances and which herbs work for you. Here are a couple of books to start you on your way:

*Rosemary Gladstar's Medicinal Herbs* by the "mother of modern herbalism" and *Herbal Remedies for Dummies* by Christopher Hobbs tell you how to harvest and prepare your own herbal teas, tinctures, and salves. (Don't be fooled by the "Dummies" title: Christopher Hobbs is a fourth-generation herbalist and well respected in the field.)

Another way to connect directly with medicinal herbs is to cook with them. "Let your food be your medicine" was the watchword of Hippocrates, the father of Western medicine. What better way than to incorporate medicinal herbs into your cuisine? There's a reason why **garlic, ginger, turmeric, cayenne** and many other herbs are so popular worldwide—and it's not just the flavor. They have anti-inflammatory, anti-bacterial, and other medicinal properties which modern science is just beginning to document. Here's a start:

*Grow Your Own Drugs:* This totally fun series of videos by British ethnobotanist James Wong will show you how to cook with medicinal herbs. The videos are jazzy, the recipes are delicious, and you can watch them online by searching for James Wong on YouTube or at **www. BBC.co.uk.**

*The Healing Power of Kitchen Herbs* by Jill Henderson and *Healing Spices: How to Use 50 Everyday and Exotic Spices to Boost Health and Beat Disease* by Bharat Aggarwal will give you new respect for the medicinal power of herbs commonly used in cooking. Dr. Aggarwal is an expert—he's doing groundbreaking research on the anticancer effect of Ayurvedic herbs at the M.D. Anderson Cancer Center in Houston.

In my own practice as a homeopath, I tend to recommend just a few single herbs over and over again. Here's the handful of single herbs which I feel everyone should know about:

**Aloe:** Aloe vera gel can be used externally for burns. You can keep a plant on the kitchen windowsill, break off a leaf and apply the gel that oozes from the leaf onto burns. Don't worry if you're like me and you can't remember to water plants. Aloe will withstand a lot of neglect. Taken internally, it heals the lining of the digestive system. George's Always Active Aloe Vera is a very effective brand, widely available in health food stores, and easy to take (or to give to your kids) because it looks and tastes like water.

**Elderberry:** Elderberry syrup is great for coughs, plus it has anti-bacterial and antiviral properties. A study done in Israel showed that elderberry extract is as effective against the flu as Tamiflu. Elderberry syrup is my go-to for coughs, and my local favorite is Maine Medicinals' Antho-Immune blend. **www.MaineMedicinals.com**. Gaia also makes a variety of great elderberry products.

**Ginkgo** is this book's "cover girl" for a reason: it's one of the most thoroughly researched herbal medicinals in hundreds of scientific studies. It helps your brain function better by improving attention, concentration, mood, energy levels, memory, and reaction time. It may even reduce the symptoms of Alzheimer's as well as a popular drug. It also increases circulation, with obvious benefits for the brain but also for poor circulation in the legs and for Raynaud's. (Caution if you're on a blood thinner, though.)

**Hawthorn** is a tonic for the heart muscle. Think about it: your heart beats approximately once per second for your entire life, without a vacation. Doesn't it make you tired just thinking about it? Hawthorn will help strengthen the heart muscle and keep it going. This is one herb whose preparation method makes a big difference in its effectiveness. A solid extract is best, for example from Gaia Herbs. It tastes like a tart berry jam, in a little jar. You can mix it with water to make a fruity drink or even spread it on toast. I like to eat it straight from the jar!

**Horsetail (Equisetum)** strengthens the bladder muscles. Great for bed-wetting kids and for women who tend to leak a little urine as they get older. You can get it, or special-order it, in your health food store. Take a dropperful twice a day in water or juice. Horsetail, like other herbs, can be mixed with juice to conceal the taste without affecting its medicinal properties.

**Milk thistle (silymarin):** This herb has the amazing ability to detoxify, heal, and restore the liver. That's so important because our livers perform dozens of different important functions in our body. (My motto: "Love Your Liver.") One of its jobs is to disarm all the toxins that come into our body through our food, water, air, medications, household cleansers, cosmetics, etc. When it can't keep up, it gets overloaded with toxins, and milk thistle comes to the rescue.

Another one of the liver's main jobs is to secrete bile, which is used to digest fats, so when the liver gets backed up, digestive problems ensue. The liver is also involved with female hormonal symptoms because it's supposed to keep breaking down estrogen, but when it gets backed up women get the symptoms of too much estrogen. It's also involved with skin conditions like psoriasis because a congested liver forces the body to use the skin as an alternate route for discharging toxins. So I often recommend a product like **Gaia Herb's Liver Cleanse** for people with toxic exposure, digestive problems, hormonal imbalance, or psoriasis.

**Ruta graveolens (rue):** Ruta grav. is a homeopathic medicine which helps to heal connective tissue such as tendons and ligaments. There's another way you can use Ruta. The homeopathic form helps *fix* tissue that's *already* torn, while the herbal form helps *strengthen* it to prevent *future* problems. For example, it could help someone who has weak ankles and tends to sprain their ankles a lot, or someone who is stressing their knees a lot with a sport with a lot of sideways moves like tennis or soccer. Ruta in tincture form can be used at the same time as the homeopathic form for extra healing power in case of injury. If your local health food store doesn't have the herbal extract, special-order the HerbPharm brand (they have it listed as Rue).

# FLOWER ESSENCES FOR
# EMOTIONAL RESCUE

Rescue Remedy, which I recommended for emergencies and emotional first aid, contains five of the 38 Bach Flower Remedies, which are like "kissing cousins" to homeopathic remedies—gentler and primarily aimed at the emotional level. Most health food stores have all 38 of these remedies, named for the British physician who wandered the English countryside following his intuition to find plants for his own healing. The information in this section is from my colleague Donna Thompson, who uses them in her counseling work.

Discovered nearly 100 years ago, these flower remedies have profound possibilities for today. For example:

**Have you lost your job?** Worried about how you will support your family? Wondering whether to move to a lower cost-of-living area and whether you can find work there? Spinning your gears instead of moving forward with a decision? Wild Oat can help you find direction and make major life choices, whether about a job, or a relationship, or moving, or buying a house. You might add Mimulus to help calm any fears, Walnut to help you adjust to change, and Clematis to help you stay grounded and focus on the issue at hand. See how easy it is to mix up a custom blend for yourself?

**Are you bogged down by negative self-talk?** Do you have all these negative, critical thoughts about yourself swirling around in your head? You might want to try Pine for negative thoughts in general, plus Crab Apple, which can help clear out toxic thoughts, mixed with White Chestnut to calm down the mind.

**How's your teenage daughter doing?** Do you just want to reach out and hug her while she's telling you to go away and leave her alone? Is she probably dealing with feeling awful about how she looks, worried the other girls don't like her, afraid to express her own individuality, like so many teenage girls today? And does your heart just break for aching about her? Maybe you could try sharing flower essences with her. Best case scenario — she would read about them and discover on her own that Larch is good for self-confidence, Centaury helps girls be more themselves and stand up for themselves, while Mimulus helps them overcome their fears.

Or maybe you might find a Flower Remedy workshop to take with her. Wouldn't that be a healing experience for both of you? Because sometimes an overworked and exhausted mom can get a little short-fused. Maybe you need some Impatiens, which helps with — surprise! — irritation and impatience.

**Do you find yourself getting angry easily?** Do you get too worked up to deal calmly with a problem? Holly might help you with those feelings and with the frustrations of dealing with moody teenagers. Donna finds that in her work as a counselor, a few drops of Holly in water and a couple of deep breaths can help people calm down almost instantaneously — so then they can focus on their healing work and dealing with their issues.

**Do you blame yourself and feel guilty for things that actually aren't your fault?** If you're carrying around a heavy weight of guilt, try some Pine so you don't feel responsible for everything. Donna remembers using it for a client who was so full of self-reproach that if Donna dropped something, the *client* would apologize.

**Do you blame others for everything bad that has happened to you?**
While it's true that some people seem to have had much more than
their share of suffering in life, if you feel that everything in your life was
caused by someone or something else, it leaves you with no leverage
to change anything. Pulling back from blaming others can be a way of
taking back your power to make positive changes in your life.

It's also a great way to stop feeding your abusers energetically, which
is what happens when you direct a lot of anger, hatred, blame, and/or
resentment towards them. If you withdraw your emotional energy, they
may lose interest and withdraw from your life. Willow is a great flower
essence for this situation.

**But what if it really *is* tough going out there in the world?** Are you
suffering setbacks? Nothing going right for you? Gentian might help
turn the situation around by giving you hope and faith so you don't
give up. Sometimes if you strengthen yourself inside, the outside world
shifts to reflect the change in you. Sounds like magic, but it isn't. It
doesn't always work, but it's worth a try.

And of course you need to *take action* to change your life at the
same time. You can't just sit at home with your Gentian essence and
expect someone to ring your doorbell with a job offer. But Gentian can
give you the motivation to go out and apply for a job, by helping you
to feel hopeful.

**Are you stuck in the past?** Brooding over past hurts or losses or in-
justices so you can't move forward in the present? Honeysuckle can help
you break free from the past. Donna remembers a client who took Honeysuckle every day for several months, until she could think about her
past without being troubled by it—or better yet, not think about it at all.

Walnut can also help you break the link with the past, which is
why it's good for any kind of life-change, like moving, graduating,
menopause, a death in the family. It helps to stabilize you and get you
through a tough time. If you use it with Chestnut Bud, it's especially
effective for learning from your past mistakes and moving on—and
with White Chestnut to break repetitive thought patterns.

Walnut is used with Clematis a lot because both are grounding. And as a bonus, it protects you against negative energies around you—something you might run into when moving into an old house or when you have to work with a real sourpuss.

**But what if you're longing for the good old days?** Honeysuckle can also help you break free from your past if you're remembering how much *better* it was, like elderly people who are so stuck reminiscing about the past that they can't be "present in the present."

## PEELING THE LAYERS OF THE ONION

Donna's favorite story about the healing power of flower essences concerns a client who was diagnosed with bipolar disorder, on multiple medications, requiring frequent hospitalizations, and who just wasn't getting better despite all the medical interventions. She consulted with Donna and used about half a dozen different combinations of flower essences, a different one each month, to "peel away the layers," as Donna put it.

"Finally she found one she felt really good on. She absolutely loved it because she felt so secure on it. She stayed on that remedy for months, and she was able to discontinue all her medications—of course, under her doctor's supervision. She stopped coming to see me, a sure sign she was doing much better. I called her several months later to check in, and she told me the good news—she no longer needed the flower essence, and she was opening her own business."

**How to Take Flower Essences**

Like herbs, flower essences work well together. They seem to support each other well and work in harmony. People often blend three to five essences to address a particular issue. Here are some ways you can take them:

- directly from the stock bottle, a few drops on the tongue
- put a few drops in water and sip on it (an easy way to blend several essences)
- in the bathtub or rubbed on pulse points, because they absorb through the skin.

As with homeopathic remedies, some people feel flower essences working right away. "As soon as I took the remedy, I felt something melting in me" is a frequent reaction reported by Donna's clients.

Others may only notice the effect after the fact. Someone close to them may point out how differently they're responding to things. Or they may look back and realize how much they've changed in the months they've been taking flower essences.

**Next Steps**

When Donna has finished using Bach Flower Essences to help a client with emotional issues, she finds they often need one of the Perelandra Rose Group essences. This family of flower essences has a different quality, Donna reports, and her clients agree. "They feel like swallowing beads of light," Donna says. "They work on a higher, more spiritual level. They take you to the soul level."

To choose among the Perelandra Rose Group essences, you'll need to explore the wealth of information on the Perelandra website or use the Perelandra Kinesiology Testing Technique which you'll also find there (**www.Perelandra-Ltd.com**).

## For Further Exploration

You can find the Bach Flower Essences in any health food store, usually accompanied by a pamphlet with a couple of sentences about each one. But Donna says the flower essences are too subtle and complex to be limited to these short descriptions, and it's better to go straight to a book about them if you're interested. Here are her favorites:

- *Advanced Bach Flower Therapy* by Gotz Blome, MD. This book comes complete with descriptions of the essences, typical symptoms for each, typical effects, how to combine them for specific problems, and a therapeutic index.
- *The Encyclopedia of Bach Flower Therapy* by Mechthild Scheffer, which will inspire you with its beautiful photographs of the flowers and empower you by teaching a self-test for figuring out your flower essence(s).

For more about the Perelandra essences, see *Behaving as if the God In All Life Mattered* and *The Perelandra Essences*, by Machaelle Small Wright, the discoverer and developer of these special essences. Available, along with the essences, from **www.Perelandra-Ltd.com**.

## Orchid Essences

My personal favorites are the Living Tree Orchid Essences made from these stunningly beautiful and unique flowers, each of which seems to have a personality and a power all its own. The healing attributes of each essence seem to "match the personality" of the flower. Gorgeous photos at **www.HealingOrchids.com**. The American distributor is **www.SouthernHerb.com**.

## THE ANGST OF ADOLESCENCE

This is from the mother of two teenage daughters whom Donna treated with flower essences. Although it's in a different format than the other stories in the book, I've kept it just as the mother wrote it because it is such a beautiful example of a loving, open, respectful, and supportive relationship between a parent and teenagers. Here is how she answered my question as to how the flower essences helped her daughters.

**The remedies introduced them to the world of energy medicine:** Conversations about the remedies are an excellent way to talk about the mind/body and head/heart connection.

**They became more self-aware/more aware of their emotions:** In the process of talking about what they needed support for from the Bach Remedies, they became expert at naming their stressors and associating them with how that made them feel. The conversation became an amazing opportunity to educate them about the importance of their emotions as a signaling system for what they needed to feel balanced and whole, and what it was specifically that was making them feel stressed and "off." Also we talked about the importance of acknowledging emotions so that they could be processed, allowed to move through so they didn't create blockages. In the Bach system there really are no "negative" emotions, and that was important for them to understand. Emotions are just emotions. Since there is so much in the culture that negates the importance of living from the heart and the gut, it gave them a way to get in touch with what happens when you don't listen.

One of the things that adolescents feel most acutely is their "difference." It's easy for them to think that there is something "wrong" with them, that no one else feels the way they do. Conversations about what they need normalize what they're feeling.

**They felt supported:** For all of us, knowing what we want or what we "should" do to feel better and actually being able to change our behavior or shift the way we look at our experience, are two different things. While taking the remedies, they could actually see and experience the subtle shifts and changes that helped them feel better and supported the changes they wanted to make.

**They felt empowered to be participants in the healing process:** By learning how to reflect on their situation, state their needs, and then actually take the remedies, they were active participants, not just doing what some expert told them to. They also become really sensitive to when they need a different remedy, when they're "done" with a particular remedy, and when another issue arises in their awareness that they want to address. My daughters have taken remedies for over ten years and they still ask for them and know when it's time to ask for their support.

**They felt heard:** A caring adult was actually sitting with them and listening to what they had to say. Their emotional life was acknowledged as important.

The process used to determine appropriate remedies translates to the rest of their life. Having the awareness to "read" what's going on in your electric body, what signals your emotions are sending about the stress in your life, asking for support, and looking for ways to restore balance are invaluable skills for life.

# CELL SALTS FOR GENTLE MENDING AND STRENGTHENING

These "energized minerals" give us the best of both worlds. Also known as tissue salts, they act as both nutritional supplements and natural medicines. The most basic minerals that the body needs are paired in twelve combinations, then "potentized" (made more powerful) through the same process used for homeopathic medicines.

Minerals are normally hard for your body to absorb. Imagine little rocks going through your digestive system and not interacting with much along the way, so they tend to come out the other end.

Put these same minerals through a dilution-and-energizing process, though, and they're highly absorbable. In fact the little soft tablets, the size of a baby aspirin, melt in your mouth.

Something else happens in the process. The minerals have now become informational blueprints or templates which remind the body how to *absorb* that mineral, *send* it where it's needed, and *use* it properly. The minerals become "teachers" for your body's healing energy.

Think about calcium for your bones, for example. How does your body know where to put the calcium? How does it know what *shape* a bone should be? And how does it know where the *edge* of the bone is supposed to be—in other words, when to stop depositing the calcium?

Sometimes the body gets it wrong and makes extra bone where it's not supposed to be. This is called a bone spur, and it's really painful. Or it can deposit calcium into little gravelly bits in the joints—ouch! Or the body may harden it into kidney stones—ouchee ouchee!

So it's tricky for the body to deposit calcium exactly into the outline of where bones are supposed to be. But the problem gets even more complicated because bones are constantly in flux. The body is constantly depositing calcium into the bones and constantly taking it out. Bones are like the body's ATM machine for depositing, saving, and withdrawing calcium.

So having strong bones is about much more than getting enough calcium in your diet. You might eat enough calcium but it might not be absorbed. Or you might take calcium in pill form, but if it's calcium carbonate, not much of it will be absorbed. Or your body might absorb the calcium and send it to the wrong place, like a bone spur.

So this is a long way 'round to explain why something as simple and innocuous as a cell salt can have such a profound effect on your body. People often ask me, "Will homeopathic remedies work even if you don't believe in them?" The short answer is "Yes, but they won't work if you don't take them—and you're more likely to take them if you have confidence that they can work." I've taken a little detour to enhance your confidence in these gentle yet powerful cell salts.

The humble little cell salts, which deserve pride of place in the natural medicine cabinet for everyday use, are too often overlooked. They are not even available in most health food stores. But it's easy to see why. They are so inexpensive ($8.95 for 500 tablets—how could something that cheap do anything?), so bland in their packaging (twelve little bottles with indistinguishable Latin names,) and so diverse in their benefits that it would be hard to know where to start if you wanted to brag about each one on its label.

So even if they make it into a store, they tend to sit meekly on the shelf, the Cinderella of supplements, with their easily-confused names and labels that look like they are relics from a 19th century apothecary.

Waiting for you to discover them and say, "Wow! Where have you been all my life, little friends?"

## Ferrum phos.

Here's the biggest wow—Ferrum phos. Every natural medicine cabinet has to have this cell salt on hand because when you need it, it's too late to buy it. This is the "nip it in the bud" remedy for any infectious illness. You use it the day *before* you or your child gets sick.

Do you have to be psychic to know when you're about to get sick? No! Just pay attention to your body. You feel low-energy, laggard, and listless. Maybe you have a mild fever or a little scratchy feeling in the back of your throat.

It's even easier to tell with kids. You know the look—they're "off their feed," with no interest in food or their favorite activities. They just want to lie on the couch, and their forehead might feel a little warm. Maybe their eyes are glassy or their cheeks are a bit flushed.

But there are no actual symptoms yet, like sneezing or coughing or a runny nose. This is the perfect time for Ferrum phos. Suck on two tablets, three times a day. Kids love them because they taste sweet.

Note that cell salts come in a special potency, 6x, which does not mean six times a day. It refers to the strength. Or your store may have them in a 12x potency. The difference is not that important.

What is important, though, is that these same remedies also come in a 30c potency, typically in the "blue tubes" in a large plexiglas dispenser in your store. So if you ask for Ferrum phos., you're likely to get a "blue tube" of Ferrum phos. 30c.

What's the difference? It's widely believed in homeopathy that as remedies are potentized more (and their "numbers go up" from 6 or 12 to 30 and even higher) they can affect your mind and emotions. The 6x potency is pretty much aimed at the physical body. It's also so mild that even the most sensitive person is unlikely to have a temporary worsening of symptoms ("aggravation") which can occasionally be part of the healing journey with homeopathy.

So cell salts are great for beginners because you really can't go wrong with them. On the other hand, you might not feel them working because they are so mild. They might chug along, like Ferrum phos. gradually helping you with anemia.

**Nutritional and medicinal uses.** Remember that cell salts are both nutritional and medicinal? Nutritional because they're more easily absorbed and assimilated as basic building blocks than ordinary mineral supplements . . . medicinal because they "teach" your body's healing energy just as homeopathic medicines do.

So Ferrum phos. has a great medicinal use—warding off colds, flus, and the common childhood illnesses—plus a major nutritional use. Can you guess? Does the word "ferrum" remind you of iron? Yes, Ferrum phos. acts like an iron supplement if you have anemia. It brings the body a little iron, and more importantly, it helps you absorb iron from your food and supplements. (Add the cell salt Calc. phos. and it will work even better.)

**Quick tips for iron supplementation.** First of all, do you need it? Iron used to be included in all multivitamins, but now there's a concern that too much could be dangerous. Women who get heavy periods (and anyone else who loses a lot of blood) are the most likely to need extra iron.

In this case, or if you've been diagnosed with anemia, consider Ferrum phos. plus an herbal iron supplement like Floradix. The body likes to get iron in herbal form because the digestive system is all set up to absorb iron from food, and herbs are basically food. The total amount of iron on the label will not look like much compared to the iron in a conventional supplement. But in my health food store, customers with anemia had great results with Floradix, as demonstrated by before-and-after blood tests, just because the iron was so well absorbed.

If you would rather take iron in pill form, take any kind *except* ferrous sulphate, which "ironically" is the kind most often recommended by doctors. Ferrous sulphate is the *only* kind of iron that is constipating.

No matter what kind of iron supplement you take, add Ferrum phos. the cell salt too, in order to help absorb it.

If you're not sure whether you need extra iron, take Ferrum phos. *instead* of an iron supplement. The cell salt is totally safe because the actual amount of iron is so small, and it works mainly by teaching your body to reach out and grab iron from your food. If your body doesn't need iron, it will tune out the message.

**Are you anemic?** Pull your lower eyelid out so you can see the pink membrane inside your eyelid and under your eye. The blood vessels are close to the skin there. Is it rosy? You're probably good to go! Pale and washed out? Could be trouble. Ideally, get your blood tested for your iron levels, and learn what your eyelids look like when you're low in iron compared to when your iron levels are normal.

## Nat. mur.

Okay, so Ferrum phos. could be your #1 friend among the twelve tissue salts. Here's my second favorite: **Nat. mur.**, short for Natrum muriaticum. It's just sodium chloride, or simple table salt. How can such a common substance have such a profound effect on your health? Doesn't make sense, does it?

But think about it. If you eat too much salt, you tend to retain water. But salt can also be used to dry things out. Salt affects the flow of water in and out of our cells, one of the most primordial functions of our body. Too much water and we feel puffy and fat—our ankles swell up, our rings don't fit. Too little water and we feel dried out and exhausted. We may not be aware of it, but our whole body, especially our brain, needs enough water to function properly. When each cell of our body is holding the proper amount of water, the beneficial effect is multiplied billions and trillions of times.

When that's not happening, many many things can go wrong, and we can't function or feel our best. That's why a simple tissue salt like Nat. mur. can have so many different uses. I'll tell you the main reason I recommend it to my clients, though: water retention or excessive dryness, like dry eyes, dry mouth, dry skin.

Does it make sense now that the same humble little mineral blend can help equally well for too much water or too little water? Conventional medicines tend to have a one-way effect because they are designed to make a specific symptom go away—like the jiggler valve on the pressure cooker described on page 197—and sometimes they overshoot their mark, creating a new imbalance, new symptoms. Homeopathic medicines often work to restore *homeostasis,* or the optimal balance in the body, by increasing something that's too low or reducing something that's in excess. They work with the natural intelligence of the body.

These Nat. mur. conditions give us a great example of how you can benchmark your own symptoms. You know whether your rings fit and whether you can get your feet into your shoes. Plus you can see in the mirror whether you have puffy bags under your eyes. Empower yourself—get to know your body!

---

## A CELL SALT TO THE RESCUE IN HAITI

Homeopaths Without Borders goes to sites of natural disasters all over the world, not only to treat the victims but also to teach the local doctors and furnish clinics with books and remedy kits. When they went to Haiti following the earthquake, they found babies at death's door from starvation. They mixed Nat. mur. with water and gave it in a dropper to the babies to rehydrate them—plus the sugar in the tablets gave a little nutrition. It was not as good as an electrolyte drink, but these drinks were in short supply, and the Nat. mur. rehydration formula was the next best thing. And for people sensitive to the emotional healing effects of cell salts, Nat. mur. would help soothe their grief.

---

## Calc. phos. and Calc. fluor.

My next top favorites among the 12 cell salts are **Calc. phos.** and **Calc. fluor.** (or to use their full-length names, Calcarea phosphorica and Calcarea fluorica—see why we use their nicknames?). Remember the question of how the body knows where bones are supposed to be? Calc.

phos. and Calc. fluor. are the "calcium supplements" among the cell salts, reminding the body to lay down healthy bone right inside the blue-print for bones. Each has a specialty: Calc. phos. says "Here's where the bone is supposed to go," while Calc. fluor. says, "Not here! Not here!"

That's right—Calc. phos. teaches the body to deposit calcium within the outline provided by the "bones template," whereas Calc. fluor. teaches it to break down calcium where it's not supposed to be. Can you imagine? You may actually be able to dissolve a bone spur or kidney stone with Calc. fluor.

Maybe not in every case, but why not try? Give it a couple of months and $10 worth of Calc. fluor. It won't hurt, and you just might be able to avoid surgery. You know the best thing about this approach? If your body has a tendency to create bone spurs, one surgery can't prevent future bone spurs, whereas your little friend Calc. fluor. just might.

**Top uses for Calc. phos., the bone builder:**
- osteoporosis and osteopenia, plus situations in which new bone is being created:
  - pregnancy, while the mom needs calcium to create a whole new set of bones for the new baby inside her
  - breastfeeding, when the mom's calcium may be depleted to provide for the baby's fast-growing bones
  - growing children, especially during growth spurts—it can even help with growing pains
  - mending broken bones, along with Symphytum (pages 91 and 205)
- osteochondritis—a kind of growing pain in teenagers' bones
- teething—it can help the new teeth push through the gums
- mental stress, especially kids studying for exams, and headaches from studying too much
- recovering from an illness like a cold or flu.

**Top uses for Calc. fluor., the "out-of-place bone dissolver":** Calc. fluor. is used not only to dissolve bone spurs, but also for other places calcium has hardened (notably kidney stones) and for softening other tissues that are too hard, like "indurated"(stony-feeling) glands, ganglion cysts, and lumps on bones from injuries ("bone bruises"). It has even been known to help with cataracts.

It affects the "elastic" tissues, ones that are supposed to "give a little." This includes arteries and veins, so it makes sense that Calc. fluor. may help with high blood pressure (if it's partly caused by stiffened arteries, Calc. fluor. may help relax them) and also with overly-lax veins such as varicose veins and hemorrhoids. (Did you know that hemorrhoids are simply varicose veins of the anus?)

There are many factors that can affect high blood pressure and hemorrhoids, so it's unlikely that Calc. fluor. alone will solve these problems. But it definitely can be part of the mix.

## The Phosphorus Salts to Soothe the Nerves

The nervous system, including the brain, depends on the mineral phosphorus to work well, so the five cell salts containing phosphorus can have a wonderful effect on a frazzled nervous system. If you're a student cramming for exams, or if you work on a computer all day, you may end up with "brain fag" (as opposed to "brain fog." "Brain fag" means a tired brain, "brain fog" means confusion, and if you have both at once, you're in trouble.)

If you feel jittery or drained, or feel like you just can't stuff one more piece of information into your tired brain, try **Kali phos.**, the specific cell salt best for brain fag and frazzled nerves. It's also great for that "tired and wired" feeling when you can't sleep because you're so exhausted, usually after mental work or mental strain.

Better yet for frazzled nerves, try a blend of all the phosphorus-containing cell salts, for example in **Hyland's Nerve Tonic**. If your health food store doesn't carry Nerve Tonic, they will definitely have its sister remedy, **Calms Forte**. It includes the same cell salts plus a homeopathic dilution of several herbs which have been used for hundreds of years to calm the nerves and promote sound sleep. So it can be used during the day for anxiety and at night for insomnia.

## A Safe Natural Sedative

I used to own a health food store near Harvard University, and Calms Forte was the most popular product in my store. In this academic environment, where people were studying hard and not getting enough sleep, they would try Calms Forte and come back to buy several bottles for friends and family members because they found it worked so well for frayed nerves, anxiety, and sleepless nights.

I remember my student days, when I would stay up all night drinking coffee to finish a term paper just before the deadline. Then I would have to cram a semester's worth of reading into my brain for exams, and I wouldn't be able to get to sleep for sheer nervousness. Then the anxiety of exam day made it even worse — sitting in Harvard's Memorial Hall with marble busts of famous professors looking down on us sternly. I wish I had known about Calms Forte then!

## Nat. phos.

**When your system is too acidic:** Let's visit just one more cell salt, **Nat. phos.**, which helps maintain your body's acid-alkaline balance, which in turn is so essential for your health. Lots of things in your body are affected by the acid-alkaline balance. Just to give one example: your body is host to billions of microbes — ideally the friendly ones that help break down your food and create vitamins in your digestive system. But when your body is too acidic, the unfriendly microbes flourish and beat out the good guys. These unfriendly ones include candida, as in vaginal yeast infections and lots of other problems from indigestion to brain fog. Another example: too much acidity can lead to indigestion with acid belching, or baby burps with a sour smell.

So how does our system get overly acidic? Too much meat, dairy products, coffee, sugar, alcohol, soda, processed foods, and stress. Sound like our modern American lifestyle? Yes it does, and overly acidic systems create huge health problems in this society. If this sounds like your diet, try Nat. phos. and see if you feel better. It can help with indigestion, parasites, and candida symptoms like vaginitis.

Many kids get worms at some point. People in the natural healing professions feel that best way to get rid of parasites like worms is to change the environment so they no longer feel welcome. Nat. phos. creates the alkaline environment that can repel worms and other parasites.

If Nat. phos. doesn't help, you may need to reduce your acid-causing factors. There's only so much a cell salt can do if your lifestyle is directly antithetical to your health.

## The Rest of the Gang

It's a funny thing about cell salts—I use half of them a lot, and the others hardly ever. Here's a quick trip through the ones I rarely use. One of them might be perfect for you.

**Calc. sulph.:** mostly for infections with creamy yellow pus that are slow to heal, like abscesses, cysts, Bartholin cysts—honestly, things I rarely see in my practice.

**Kali mur.:** to re-absorb fluid in the ear, like in swimmer's ear or an ear infection. Isn't this an amazing concept? It's like Calc. fluor. teaching your body to break down and re-absorb a bone spur. Here you are telling your body to take the fluid in the ear and re-absorb it. Otherwise it could be there for a long time. Annoying!

**Mag. phos.** is used for cramping, but I usually use Mag. phos. 30c, the fully potentized homeopathic remedy, because it's stronger and faster-acting. Use the cell salt Mag. phos. 6x, though, if you need it right away and don't have the 30c on hand. Also if you tend to get cramps frequently, Mag. phos. 6x may work gradually over time to reduce them.

**Kali sulph.:** like Calc. sulph., Kali sulph. is associated with late-stage infections with creamy yellow discharges. It's used for skin conditions like eczema and psoriasis, and also for sinusitis, asthma, and rattling mucus in the chest. If you have a chronic condition like this, use Kali sulph. to tide you over while you're looking for a professional homeopath or naturopath for deeper, more lasting healing.

**Nat. sulph.:** found in the fluid between cells, Nat. sulph. can help clear out this fluid along with the toxins that can accumulate there. It's also supportive when someone has liver problems.

**Silicea:** this one is huge. I should have included it with my faves. We already talked about it in the Splinters section, page 123. (For some reason the cell salt is spelled Silicea.) It strengthens thin or brittle hair and nails, or skin that doesn't heal easily, like the fragile skin of elderly people. This is a great addition to your natural beauty kit as well as your medicine cabinet.

    Caution: this is the same Silica that can push out foreign objects like splinters (good) or pacemakers (bad). Never use Silica in any potency if the person has an implanted medical device. Luckily it doesn't seem to affect IUDs or fillings in your teeth, though (based on reports from my fellow homeopaths).

**Bioplasma:** I saved the best for last. If you want to get the benefit of all twelve cell salts as a nutritional supplement, you can get them in a blend called Bioplasma. Lots of people feel a benefit from this blend, probably because our soils are so depleted in minerals from our commercial farming practices.

    Remember, though, that Bioplasma only covers some of the main minerals, not the trace minerals. Sea vegetables like nori (you know it and love it, it's the thin crispy wrapping for sushi) are a great source of the dozens of trace minerals that our bodies need in tiny amounts.

And if you want one cell salt to address a specific symptom, it's better to take it in isolation because you want your body to get the message from that particular medicine. It's like trying to learn a song—better to have just one person sing the song to you over and over, instead of twelve people each singing a different song at the same time and blurring the message. For medicinal purposes, the cell salts shape-shift from *nutritional supplements* to energy-based, informational *medicines*, and in this case, the message is more important than the miniscule amount of "stuff" (the actual mineral) in the cell salt.

## Using the Cell Salts

If a store has them, they will be on a shelf in a set of twelve near the homeopathic remedies. They will probably be labeled 6x (that's the strength; it doesn't mean to take them 6 times a day). Some stores have them in the 12x potency. These potencies can be used interchangeably.

A typical dosage is two pellets three times a day. But that's just an average. Use them more frequently if the symptoms are urgent or severe, less often if you're dealing with a chronic condition that has become like background music.

## Do Cell Salts Have Emotional Effects?

Cell salts mostly work on the physical plane, unlike fully potentized homeopathic remedies (ones whose numbers end in "c" like 6c, 30c and especially the higher numbers or potencies). These fully potentized remedies are like a chord in music with notes in several octaves (or in this case, on the physical, emotional, mental, energetic, and behavioral levels).

I can only remember a single instance of a client taking a cell salt (in this case Nat. mur. for excessive dryness) who reported an unexpected emotional effect, the resolution of a chronic grief state. She was one of the most hypersensitive clients I've ever worked with, so it was no surprise that she was the only one to have an emotional reaction.

Well-known homeopath Miranda Castro, who is an expert on cell salts, reports an emotional healing with Nat. mur.—in the case of a cat! This story is from our companion volume on natural remedies for animals. It's so good I'll repeat it here.

## THE TALE OF THE SULKY CAT

Miranda tells of arriving at a friend's house to teach a class on cell salts and finding the friend's cat by the front door in a little alcove, its head pointing into the shadows. The cat had been there for several days, head down, refusing to come out or to eat. If the cat were a person, you would say she looked depressed.

Apparently this behavior began when a new kitten arrived and the older cat seemed to feel it had lost its special position, as everyone in the family began doting on the adorable kitten.

When Miranda got to the cell salt **Nat. mur.**, she described its emotional aspect as silent grief, often with resentment or bitterness at a loss. The person who needs it is likely to suffer in silence rather than crying hysterically (as someone would who needed Ignatia, for example), and they may refuse to eat.

The whole class gasped, "The cat!" The cat's mum went and gave it Nat. mur. (It wasn't easy—she had to force a tablet into the cat's cheek pouch.)

Half an hour later the cat walked through the open front door, through the living room where the class was being held, and went straight to the basket where the kitten was sleeping. She climbed into the basket, curled up around the kitten, and went to sleep.

She was absolutely fine after that. She and the kitten became fast friends. A single dose of Nat. mur. helped her to recover from the grief of losing her special place in the family's affections.

---

### For More Information

Miranda Castro's DVD set, *The Twelve Fabulous Cell Salts*, is the best introduction, available from **www.MirandaCastro.com**.

Or if you'd rather read a book, try *Natural Healing with Cell Salts* by Skye Weintraub.

And if you really want to have fun with cell salts, check out *Facial Diagnosis of Cell Salt Deficiencies* by David Card. It's full of color pictures illustrating how a deficiency of each cell salt can show up in skin color and texture and many other facial features. You can use it to figure out your friends' cell salt needs — it's totally safe, and if it works, they'll be pleasantly surprised.

# HOMEOPATHIC MEDICINES: A STARTER SET

## Arnica

This is the best single remedy for every medicine cabinet and gym bag, along with its friends **Topricin** or **Traumeel,** the topical ointments.

If you can remember these three key symptoms, you'll know how to use it:

∾ **bruised**
∾ **soft tissue trauma**
∾ **"I'm fine! Leave me alone!"**

It's perfect for those times when people have been injured and the endorphins (natural painkillers) come out and they **don't feel pain**, but you know they're hurt.

It also works for a variety of conditions where there hasn't been an actual blow, but the person feels bruised, sore, or beaten up, for example after surgery or even during the flu.

So here's a list of what it's useful for. You don't have to memorize the list, just remember those three keys to Arnica:

∾ after childbirth for mother and baby, especially if the baby has a bruise on its head
∾ black eyes
∾ bruises

- concussion, while waiting for appropriate medical help
- dental extractions (see page 129 for the remedies, page 211 for instructions)
- nosebleeds, especially after a blow to the nose
- sore muscles, pulled muscles
- sports injuries, sprains, and strains
- surgery (see pages 129 and 211).

## ARNICA ON THE CATWALK

Recently the *New York Times* ran an article on the top fashion models and designers using Arnica. "Arnica gel is the best thing you can do for bruises," according to Diane Von Furstenberg, quoted in the article, and apparently Phillip Lim uses it to remove puffiness under his eyes before fashion shows.

The article got some of the basic information about Arnica totally wrong, though. It quoted a dermatologist who uses *herbal* Arnica topically and cautions against taking it orally because it could be toxic. Remember the difference between herbs and homeopathy? Herbs have actual stuff in them, while homeopathy conveys information and can never build up to toxic levels because there's not enough material substance in it.

Soccer superstar David Beckham uses Arnica, as do many of the top sports teams and athletes in Europe. American athletes are starting to catch on as well. The *New York Times* article referred to the head fitness coach for the US Men's National Soccer Team introducing its use in 2002. Read about the top celebrities and athletes using homeopathy in Dana Ullman's fascinating book *The Homeopathic Revolution*.

## THE LITTLE GIRL AND THE PHARMACIST

I was helping a friend babysit his four-year-old daughter while his wife was out for the evening. His little girl ran into the living room, skidded on the rug, tripped over the dog, and banged her forehead on the corner of the piano bench. Ouch!

Her forehead started to swell visibly and she soon had a goose-egg the size of half a baseball. We gave her Arnica and the goose-egg disappeared as quickly as it had appeared, before her mom came home, to our immense relief. Since she had no signs of a concussion, her dad felt comfortable waiting until the next day to take her to the doctor, who said she was fine.

A pharmacist friend decided to do an experiment when she got a large bruise. She rubbed Arnica cream on half of it, which went away immediately, leaving the other untreated half to turn shades of green and purple for a week.

You might want to try this too. Do your own science experiment on yourself!

## Arsenicum

Okay, let's get it over with—how can you use a poison as a medicine? It really is made from arsenic, but it's so diluted that the trace amounts ('nanoparticles') can't be detected by conventional methods (see page 212). Apparently they behave differently than full strength arsenic, conveying information to the body's healing energy—information about how to fend off the symptoms that arsenic would cause in full strength, symptoms like burning diarrhea and extreme exhaustion.

Your body knows how to be healthy. It just gets thrown off base by different blows or shocks to the system, which can be physical or emotional.

The remedy gives the body information that reminds it of its natural healthy state. It's like calling in the piano tuner when your piano is out of tune. You wouldn't start with a hammer and saw, would you? Save powerful medical interventions for when they're really needed.

Anyway, getting back to Arsenicum, it will become one of your best remedy friends! Here are your key concepts for Arsenicum:

- **anxious and fretful about** survival issues like health, money, and having a roof over your head; also about things being out of place
- **extreme exhaustion** "out of proportion" (like, why would someone need to stay in bed for a week with a cold?)
- **watery, drippy nasal discharge** ("nose running like a faucet") causing chapping of the skin under the nose ("red mustache")
- **burning sensation**, for example with diarrhea
- **worse after midnight** (including insomnia), with a restlessness that makes the person get out of bed and drive you crazy, if it's your spouse.

Once you know these key concepts, you can use it for so many things:

- acute anxiety
- colds and flu
- other infectious conditions: coughs, sore throats, conjunctivitis
- diarrhea, especially travelers' diarrhea and food poisoning
- hay fever with that watery nasal discharge
- headaches
- insomnia
- mouth sores with a burning sensation
- nausea and vomiting
- shingles.

Each of these conditions could require a different remedy, though. Look for the typical Arsenicum tiredness, fretfulness and restlessness to make sure you have a good match.

### THE NEAT FREAK HUSBAND

A friend called because her husband had a cold. These phone calls can be tricky because I can't observe the person myself. The most helpful information for finding a good homeopathic remedy is often the most unusual symptom (because that helps narrow down the choice), but people usually report the most common symptoms (which are the least helpful).

This was a typical example. I asked her for his symptoms and she said, "He's lying in bed. He's sneezing. His nose is running." Okay, so far, those symptoms could match about a dozen different remedies! "What is he doing?" I asked, trying to narrow down the choice. "He's ordering me around, telling me to clean up the room." Bingo! This behavior matched the fussy neatness of someone needing Arsenicum, plus their tendency to be bossy.

Did it work? I never found out. Typically people only call back if they feel worse!

## Calendula

Anytime the skin is broken or cut, **Calendula** is your best friend. It does several important things:
- **knits together** the two sides of a cut
- helps **prevent infection**
- **reduces pain**
- **prevents scarring**

Calendula works well in herbal form (in other words, when it's present in full strength, not homeopathically diluted). Your health food store will have a variety of creams, lotions, and sprays with Calendula tincture. The spray is especially good for applying to a very tender area, say a burn, where you don't want to smear something on it.

Calendula works even better in homeopathic pellet form, which you'll probably have to special-order because stores don't usually carry it. Taking it internally works especially well if the person needs it over a large area of the body.

You also have the flexibility of dissolving a few pellets in water and applying it directly to the wound and/or soaking the bandage in Calendula water. (If you've had surgery, wait until your doctor says it's okay to use a wet dressing.) You'll probably get quicker results if you use it both ways (taking it internally and applying it topically).

So you'll probably start off with a topical (surface) application of Calendula, but in the long run, if you want a well-equipped natural medicine cabinet, it would be wise to get homeopathic Calendula in pellet form (page 202 for a supplier).

### The Grandma Who Hopped Over the Bed Rails

I've had some dramatic results with **Arnica** and **Calendula** as part of the pre- and post-surgery protocol described on page 211.

One of my students used it for her mother, who was in her 80s and was in the hospital for bowel resection surgery. In other words, her abdomen would be cut open and part of her bowel removed, then the parts stitched together—so it involved lots of cutting, a very painful kind of surgery.

I remember from my nursing school days that part of our job was to try to get patients up out of bed after surgery and walking a few steps, on a schedule prescribed by the doctor . . . and I remember how hard it was to do that, especially with elderly people. It would be so painful for them to move, they just wanted to lie in bed and conserve their energy.

Do you know, this elderly lady, the day after this painful abdominal surgery (according to her daughter) shocked her nurses by sitting up in bed unaided, climbing over the bed rails and walking to the bathroom by herself!

One of my clients told me a similar story.

Her mother, sadly, needed a double mastectomy; my client asked me for the surgery remedies for her mom.

After an operation like this, patients typically get pain medication on a schedule, plus they can also dispense extra pain medication when they need it.

The nurses were amazed that even after having both breasts removed (can you imagine how painful that would be?) this woman did not use any of her additional pain medication.

---

I've heard many similar stories, from my clients and students, of using the surgery remedies and having the surgeon comment afterwards that it was her or his "best work" because the incision healed so beautifully with minimal pain and scarring.

Unfortunately, none of the patients told the surgeon that they had used homeopathic remedies. I hope that you will share with your doctor the results you get from using these remedies. It will help doctors to become more comfortable with natural healing.

## Gelsemium

This is our top medicine for flu and many viral conditions when the person feels totally flattened and drained of energy. You can often tell when someone needs it because they are so exhausted, their eyelids are drooping.

It's also a great remedy for "hearing bad news" when the person reacts by going numb. Instead of crying, they shut down. They may feel like their brain freezes up and they can't think of what to do (that "deer in the headlights" feeling). And they may feel so totally drained of energy that they can hardly move (that "just got run over by a truck" kind of totally flattened feeling). So they look like they've got the flu, but it may be all emotional.

**Gelsemium** is your best friend for this kind of reaction. Here are your key concepts:

- **dizzy, drowsy, droopy, dopy**
- **anticipation anxiety** with diarrhea
- **"hearing bad news"** and reacting with emotional numbness.

So here are lots of ways to use Gelsemium:

- anxiety before exams, performing on stage, medical procedures or dental work
- anxiety before the vet, for pets
- diarrhea
- fever and chills
- flu
- insomnia when you can't sleep even though you're exhausted, or from anxiety, or mental overwork
- vertigo (remember the "dizzy" symptom: you might feel dizzy with the flu, or you might have vertigo by itself).

## A MYSTERY FLU IN AUGUST

I was serving as a volunteer medic on a meditation retreat on Long Island. One young man asked for a remedy for what seemed to be the flu—quite odd on a sweltering August day. The typical flu symptoms were there: he felt absolutely lousy, he was totally drained of energy, and even his eyelids were droopy. I realized he needed Gelsemium but I thought that maybe he didn't actually have the flu—maybe there was something else going on. To help find a remedy that matched him, I asked what was the biggest stress in his life when he started to feel sick.

He said there was a big stress but he was sure it had nothing to do with getting the flu (which he was sure he had). He had gone into Manhattan and had not seen a hidden "No Parking/Tow Zone" sign. His car was towed and it cost him several hundred dollars in cash to get it back—money he didn't have in his account.

Well, this is a great example of "hearing bad news." First he went through the shock of thinking his car had been stolen. Then he found out that he had to fork over that cash he didn't have. To make matters worse, there was a storage fee for each day that he failed to pick up the car, so the cost kept going up and up while he tried to scrounge up the cash.

His body reacted to this series of "hearing bad news" as if it were punched down, like a boxer that gets punched down again before he can stagger to his feet. This kind of blow can make people react in a Gelsemium kind of way. So that's why he seemed to have flu symptoms in August. He perked right up after a dose of Gelsemium.

## Hypericum

When you injure yourself in a nerve-rich area like a fingertip, toe, or lip, use **Hypericum**, the homeopathic medicine for nerve injuries.

Another nerve-rich area is the base of the spine, so Hypericum can relieve the pain when someone slips and falls right on their "tush." Remember to go to your chiropractor if it was a serious fall.

Another injury to a nerve-rich area: a tear or an episiotomy (a planned incision to allow for more stretching) during childbirth. Ouch, what a painful area! Hypericum will help.

Hypericum is also great for shooting pains which are likely to be along the path of a nerve. For example, when people describe pain going from a tooth into the jaw along a path like a thin line or a thin thread, they may get great relief from Hypericum.

It might even work for sciatica, which is pain along the sciatic nerve, especially if the person feels the pain shooting along the nerve (which goes down the leg). It's worth a try, but there are lots of other remedies for sciatica. So if Hypericum doesn't work, please see Dr. Asa Hershoff's *Homeopathy and Musculoskeletal Healing* or seek help from a chiropractor or a professional homeopath (see page 238).

Here are the two main concepts for Hypericum:

∽ **crushed nerves**
∽ **nerve pain** like pins and needles, or shooting along the path of a nerve.

Here are some situations when you might use it:

∽ when you hit your finger (a nerve-rich area) with a hammer
∽ when you hit or badly cut your lip
∽ a piercing on the lip, tongue or other tender area
∽ a tear or incision in the vaginal area during childbirth
∽ a puncture wound
∽ when you fall and hurt your tailbone, or for an injury to the spine, while you are on the way to professional care
∽ pain in the root of a tooth especially if it feels like a thin thread of pain going into the jaw

∾ phantom limb pain after an amputation

∾ sciatica, if the pain shoots along the path of the nerve.

## Ignatia

∾ Your teenage daughter's boyfriend just dumped her.

∾ Your tween is the victim of mean, slanderous gossip being instant-messaged around the class.

∾ Your best friend's husband just left her for another woman.

∾ You just got the phone call you've been dreading—an elderly parent has passed away.

∾ Your teenager has had a car accident and is in the hospital.

∾ Your boss just humiliated you in front of everyone at a staff meeting by blaming you for something to save face for himself.

Homeopaths call these situations **"hearing bad news,"** and when someone gets sick (physically or emotionally) as a result, we say they are "never well since hearing bad news." What do all these situations have in common? **Sudden strong emotions,** whether grief or fear or shame or anger over injustice.

Homeopathy can help here too. It can't change the situation, but it can give you the inner strength, the poise, and the presence of mind to deal with it in a mature way.

**Ignatia** is your best friend in this situation, for sudden emotional upsets and stormy emotions in people of any age. It's especially great for teenagers. "Sighing and sobbing" are the watchwords for this remedy. People who need it show their tumultuous emotions by sobbing hysterically or heaving a sigh.

So you already know three key words for Ignatia:

∾ **sighing** (maybe from a feeling of a heavy weight on the chest)

∾ **sobbing**

∾ **stormy emotions.**

Here are a couple more, then you know the whole remedy:

∾ **psychosomatic symptoms** (physical symptoms that are really an expression of strong emotions)

∾ **cramps and spasms** (muscle cramps or a cramping sensation).

So let's put these concepts together and here's an overview of what you can use Ignatia for:

∾ **emotional support** in a crisis

∾ **insomnia** when upset, when "rehearsing" for a relationship problem ("I wish I told that guy off . . . next time I see him I'll . . .")

∾ any **physical symptom** caused by stormy emotions, especially ones involving cramps or spasms:

  ○ spasmodic coughing
  ○ nausea/vomiting
  ○ lump in the throat (throat muscles cramped together)
  ○ back spasms, rectal spasms, or other muscle cramps
  ○ colic in an infant, especially if the mom is upset.

### Does Ignatia Just Numb Your Grief?

"I've offered my friend some Ignatia and she says she wants to feel her emotions, she doesn't want to take a drug to numb herself to her grief."

This is an understandable reaction—actually a praiseworthy reaction—because too often in this society, people use all kinds of things to avoid feeling their feelings:

∾ alcohol or drugs (whether prescription drugs or recreational drugs),

∾ zoning out watching TV, immersing themselves in the internet, or

∾ losing themselves in a fantasy world of gaming in which they've created another identity for themselves—one that can't be touched by grief.

When these forms of entertainment are used to avoid feeling grief or other strong emotion, several unhealthy things can happen:

~ The body may find an outlet for the strong emotions in the form of **physical illness**. We homeopaths see this all the time in our professional practice.

~ A lot of **life-energy is wasted**. A lot of life-energy is going into the emotion itself, and even more into suppressing the emotion, meaning that less is available for family, career, or creativity.

~ And it's **not a good role model for children**. Kids have their little antennae out for parents who are upset or tense, and parents who numb themselves and avoid the problem are creating a not-helpful life-lesson for their kids.

So it's better to feel our painful feelings rather than numb ourselves. Ignatia and other homeopathic remedies don't numb our feelings. They strengthen the core part of ourselves, the part that is processing the grief and coping with the difficult situation.

### AN INCONSOLABLE MOTHER

I once had a client who missed her only son terribly. He had just left for college in another country, and it was dawning on her that he would probably never live at home again. So in some sense she had lost him, at least she had lost him as her little boy.

I offered her Ignatia and she refused it at first, saying she wanted to feel her feelings. She was having a hard time functioning, though, because she was crying so much, and—a sure clue to Ignatia—also sighing heavily.

Finally she took it, and was very pleased with the results. She reported, "I can grieve without sobbing and I can feel my feelings without getting hysterical." **Hysterical** is a great keyword for Ignatia.

## Kali bic.

This is the best remedy for thick sticky mucus, like when you blow your nose or cough up phlegm, and there's a long string of mucus to your mouth or nose—yuck! **Kali bic.** sounds like "bick", and we say "When mucus sticks, use Kali bic." It may not form an actual string, but the consistency will remind you of rubber cement.

Kali bic. loosens thick, sticky mucus anywhere in the body:
- in the nose
- in the sinuses
- in the ears, when you have to pop your ears, like in a plane but this time it's to clear the mucus
- mucus you can't get up from your lungs.

Because the mucus is so sticky, it's hard to dislodge it. So you'll probably need to make this remedy stronger by putting it in water (see page 208).

## Nux Vomica

Nux covers problems in the digestive tract, from heartburn to hemorrhoids, plus several others to boot. Here are your key concepts for Nux vomica:
- **digestive** problems
- **cramps** and cramping pain
- **worse from overindulging** in rich/fatty food, junk food, spicy food, alcohol
- **irritable**
- liver: anything affecting the liver such as alcohol, fatty foods, or toxins that the liver has to break down.

So here are a wide range of **digestive conditions** Nux can help with, *if* the symptoms match:

~ cramping pains in the stomach or abdomen
~ constipation, perhaps with ineffectual cramping
~ diarrhea
~ acute gallbladder attack
~ hangovers (which happen when the liver gets toxic from too much alcohol)
~ heartburn
~ hemorrhoids
~ nausea and vomiting.

It may not work if your symptoms don't match (there are other remedies for each of these conditions), but there's no harm in trying as long as you follow the guidelines on pages 204-208.

### VOMITING AFTER NUX VOMICA

This happened to me after drinking a bottle of the fermented health drink Kombucha. It's usually one of my favorite things, but maybe this bottle had not been properly prepared . . . anyway, I felt nauseous as soon as I drank it. I took some Nux vomica and instantly threw up.

I knew this must be an effect of Nux because it's the first time in 50 years that I've thrown up, so it couldn't have been a coincidence.

I concluded that my body, in its wisdom, used the information from the dose of Nux to speed up what it was trying to do anyway.

Homeopathy does not **suppress symptoms,** which means forcing symptoms to disappear while leaving the underlying problem untouched.

Suppressing symptoms is dangerous because the underlying problem has to find another way to vent itself—usually a more destructive way than before. Suppressing the body's symptoms is like blocking the little jiggler valve on top of a pressure cooker. Eventually it will explode. The body can't explode, of course, but it may find new symptoms as an outlet, and these new symptoms are usually worse than the ones that were blocked.

In my case, if I had taken an anti-vomiting drug, my body would probably have gotten rid of the offending substance through a bad case of diarrhea. Or maybe I would have gotten really sick from the spoiled food.

## Phosphorus

Phosphorus is a great remedy to have on hand for **bright red bleeding**:
- bleeding gums
- bleeding hemorrhoids
- cuts that just won't stop bleeding
- after surgery or a tooth extraction
- coughing or vomiting blood
- nosebleed
- heavy menstrual bleeding or bleeding from fibroids
- postpartum hemorrhage.

Phosphorus might stop the bleeding or help control it while you get appropriate medical help. Some people bleed more easily than others, and have a harder time getting the bleeding to stop. These people are often likely to need Phosphorus to control the bleeding.

For these people, a dose of Phosphorus can be taken preventively before surgery or a tooth extraction. See the pre- and post-surgery instructions on page 211. As a bonus, Phosphorus will also help people come out of anesthesia who usually have to be "slapped awake."

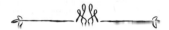

## Part Four

# HOW TO USE HOMEOPATHIC MEDICINES

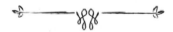

Homeopathic medicines are the most powerful natural remedies, in my experience—that's why I decided to become a homeopath after 15 years in my health food store. Oftentimes you can actually feel them working, and sometimes they seem to work instantaneously.

They are tricky, though. Sometimes they don't work, because they follow laws and principles of healing which are quite different from conventional medications. There are so many reasons why they may not work! For example, if you take too much they have a boomerang effect. More is not better when it comes to homeopathy. When the remedy starts to work, you have to stop taking it and let your body's healing energy take over.

It takes a bit of time to master homeopathy's healing principles, but it's worth it because they are powerful and gentle at the same time, non-addictive and safe to have around kids. So in this section I'll explain how to buy them and use them and the common pitfalls people tend to fall into, plus resources for learning more about them.

# BUYING HOMEOPATHIC
# MEDICINES AND
# HOW TO USE THEM

New to this? just dipping your toe in the water? You can buy these remedies as the need comes up, from any health food store, some drug stores,
and online. They typically cost about $7 for enough to last a long time.

Most people do best with a 30c potency (strength), the most
common potency in stores. A few tough cookies need their remedies
stronger, while a few hypersensitives will overreact to a 30c and will
need them milder. We're getting to that.

If you get them in a health food store, you'll probably find the
"blue tube" remedies made by Boiron in a plexiglas display case. Some
stores carry an additional line, Hylands, which comes in a square white
jar with a red cap. I have a slight preference for this brand because the
soft tablets dissolve easily in water or in a child's mouth.

If you want to get them online, I recommend getting them from
Homeopathic Educational Services, **www.Homeopathic.com**, because
the site also has so much useful information.

Ready to roll up your sleeves and really dig in? Better yet, buy a
whole kit:

∞ You'll save hundreds of dollars in the long run.
∞ You'll have them on hand if you need them in the middle of the
night.

∾ The pellets are tiny and dissolve easily in water.

∾ The kit is so compact, it's easy to travel with.

I recommend the First Aid Emergency Kit of 50 remedies from Natural Health Supply, **www.a2zhomeopathy.com.** Get them in the 30c potency (strength), the most common strength to use for home care. They come in a very compact box, handy for traveling, with hundreds of tiny pellets in each tube. You can also buy them individually.

**How to open the tube:** If you bought the typical blue tube (Boiron brand) in a store, you're probably baffled. Don't feel bad, you're in good company. Nobody can open the tube and nobody can pronounce the name. A friend of mine with a PhD bought a blue tube after reading my book and had to call me because she couldn't open it.

The plastic cap is designed so that if you hold the tube upright with the cap on the bottom, then twist the cap, the pellets will pop out one at a time. Then you can use the cap to pour them into your mouth without touching them. The first time you do this, you may need to peel off a tiny strip of paper which safety-seals the cap to the tube.

It's a clever design based on the popular belief that you shouldn't touch the pellets with your hands—but in my experience, it's an unnecessary safeguard. I've put hundreds of doses right into people's hands and they worked just fine. (I was forced to do this experiment when I was a volunteer medic on a meditation retreat in a Third World country. Everybody was sick, I ran out of my little dispensing envelopes and there was no way to buy more. So I poured the pellets into people's hands and they worked just fine.)

As for pronouncing Boiron, try "Bwa-RONH" where the last syllable has a soft throaty R—a French rolled R—and soft nasal N. Or just ask the store staff for a blue tube.

**Under the tongue?** It's widely believed that the homeopathic pellets have to go under your tongue. Actually they work when they touch mucous membranes, like your gums and cheeks, so just suck on them and roll them around in your mouth. They even work on thin skin, like your temples or the inside of your wrists. You can give them to a baby by dissolving them in water (page 209) and dabbing them on the temple.

**What about antidotes?** You may have heard that many substances can antidote (inactivate or cancel out) homeopathic medicines. Some professional homeopaths give their clients a long list of substances to avoid, such as coffee, mint, camphor, Ben-Gay or Vicks Vapo-Rub, dental work, airport x-rays, electric blankets,,, Here's the funny thing: even though many homeopaths tell their clients they can't drink coffee, if you go to a homeopathy convention you might as well open a Starbucks outlet right there in the meeting room because everybody is drinking coffee.

In my experience, these substances don't interfere with homeopathic medicines for home use. There is a long tradition in homeopathy about these antidotes, but no actual research. (We get so little money for research, we don't want to waste it on a question like this.) To be on the safe side, I simply ask clients to have a "clean mouth" which means no strong taste or odor in the mouth when they take their medicine.

---

### STOPPED AT SECURITY WITH MY BULLET BOX

My traveling kit is the Natural Health Supply kit that I recommend in this book. If you look closely at the lid, you'll see stamped in the plastic "Colt 45." That's right, it's actually a box to hold bullets. It fits the little medicine bottles perfectly. But it does tend to attract attention in an airport scanner, so I'm accustomed to being stopped.

While going through JFK recently, I was not surprised when I was asked to retrieve my "bullet box" from my carry-on for inspection. What did surprise me, though, was the reaction of the security guard when she examined it. "Those are homeopathic remedies!" she screamed at the top of her lungs. "You're not supposed to let them get x-rayed!"

I reassured her that I am indeed a homeopath and I know what I'm doing—and I congratulated her on her knowledge and her carefulness.

---

## How to Give the Remedies

**Two pellets every four hours**: typically you would give two pellets every four hours as long as the symptoms are INTENSE (the injury just happened and really hurts) then **twice a day** when the person is on the mend.

Even if the label says five pellets, you really only need two. And if it says to "take twice a day," remember that's a generic suggestion which doesn't necessarily fit your situation.

**Slow down as soon as it starts to work** because you're just trying to "get the ball rolling." Wait, let it work, and repeat again when the symptoms start to come back. This is another way in which homeopathy is quite different from conventional medicine. You know how you're supposed to finish your round of antibiotics even if you feel better? It's the opposite in homeopathy. As soon as you start to feel better, it means the momentum of healing is underway, and you need to just step back and let it keep going.

**Stop when you're totally better.** You can always take another dose if the symptoms come back.

**In a real emergency** (someone is bleeding badly, you're waiting for the medics), give as often as **every 15 minutes**.

**Keep notes!** You'll get the hang of this and it will come to seem like second nature, but in the beginning it feels like too many variables to keep track of. Always write down the date, the remedy you gave, why you gave it, and how well it worked.

## It Didn't Work! What Went Wrong?

**You didn't give enough doses:** My clients often call me to say that a remedy I recommended did not work, typically for a sick child. Then it turns out that they only gave one dose!

**It wasn't strong enough** for the person or the situation: see **Making the Remedies Stronger**, below.

**It wasn't the right remedy:** Giving a remedy is like striking a tuning fork. Another tuning fork of the same pitch will vibrate. One of a different pitch won't respond. If the remedy doesn't match your symptoms well, your body won't respond. In this book I've focused on first aid and other situations in which one remedy is likely to work. Other conditions like coughs or headaches have dozens of potential remedies. I'm saving them for my next book!

**Too soon to tell:** Maybe it's working but it's too soon to tell, like a broken bone. You wouldn't expect that to get better after just a few doses. You might not even feel less pain at that point. But Symphytum is such a good remedy for broken bones (along with its little friend the cell salt Calc. phos.), you'll just keep giving it. On the other hand, nausea can change on a dime, so if it's not responding after a few doses, you might need something else.

**Too strong, made things worse:** Maybe it actually did work but it was too strong right off the bat, and it made the symptoms *temporarily* worse. This is called an aggravation, and don't worry, not only will it wear off soon but typically the person will then feel even *better than before* the dose. These aggravations rarely happen in home-prescribing situations. But in a culture that believes "more is better," it can happen when the person is better but keeps taking more of the remedy. See "Slow Down" and "Stop" on page 204.

**It did work, by shortening the current phase:** Maybe it actually did work by moving the symptoms along to the next phase, for example changing a cold from the early stage (watery/drippy) to late stage (thick sticky mucus). When the symptoms change dramatically, you need to change the remedy—and you just made the cold a lot shorter. Congratulations!

---

### "JUST TOP IT OFF"

A friend called because she had gotten poison ivy working in her garden. I suggested she get Rhus tox., the top remedy for poison ivy. It worked after just one dose because she happens to be very sensitive to the remedies. She stopped itching, but then she decided to take one more dose "just to top it off." Big mistake! The itching came back worse than ever! I told her to take an oatmeal bath (powdered oatmeal in hot water) instead of repeating the remedy. The next day her poison ivy was really gone.

---

### Making the Remedies Stronger

The 30c potency (strength), the standard potency in health food stores, works fine for most people when given in a "dry dose" (pellets dissolved in the mouth). But sometimes you need to make the remedy stronger:

- because of the **situation** (like when you're flattened by the flu, or bleeding heavily and waiting for the ambulance)
- or because the **nature of the symptom** is hard to budge, like the

thick sticky mucus of Kali bic (page 195)

- ∾ or the **person tends to be a slow responder.** You'll find this out by experience as you treat more family members and friends. Some people usually feel remedies working as soon as they touch their mouth, while other people need a *lot* before they notice anything. In my experience, women tend to be more sensitive to their bodies, which might be why women tend to be more interested in natural healing.

- ∾ or there's something that **keeps triggering the condition** you're treating. Let's say you're sick from getting soaked and chilled. Normally you would get warm and dry, but what if you're out camping and the cold rain is relentless? (I hope you brought your remedies with you!).

To make the remedies stronger, you can:

- ∾ Give them **more frequently,** because the frequency of the dose is more important than the number of pellets in each dose. The remedy is trying to teach your body something. If you're trying to learn a song, you'll learn better from having one person sing it to you over and over (that's like repeating the remedy), rather than from having a lot of people sing it just once (which is like taking a lot of pellets in a single dose). Taking a lot of pellets at once is only a little stronger than taking a few, and it just wastes the pellets.

- ∾ Give them in water (see below.)

- ∾ If you or someone in your family consistently need remedies stronger, you can buy them in a **higher potency** (strength). The most commonly available next-higher potency is 200c, but that's a *lot* stronger. I don't recommend it for home use, especially for beginners. Natural Health Supply has the remedies in a 100c potency, a more natural next step above the 30c (**www.a2zhomeopathy.com,** look at the Homeopathic Remedies section). But please always start with 30c before trying a higher potency. You'll be surprised at how much it can do.

## Giving Remedies in Water to Make Them Stronger

Dissolving a couple of pellets in about a half cup of water, and taking it sip by sip, can make the remedies **stronger**. Doesn't make any sense, does it? The remedies are more diluted—how can they be stronger? Well, if they were only diluted, then you would be right. But they go through another process at each stage of dilution. Succussion (hard thwacking) as part of the manufacturing process apparently increases the nano-particles which are the high-tech reason why they work (page 212.)

When you dilute them in a small amount of water and stir really, really well, all of the water takes on the properties of the remedy pellet. Each sip is like a great big pellet—it touches a much bigger area. If you **swish it like mouthwash** before swallowing, it will touch even more of an area and can act even more effectively.

To make it even stronger, you can **succuss the remedy**. You'll need to have it in a small bottle rather than a glass. Hold the bottle with one hand and whack it firmly against the palm of the opposite hand. (Or you can use a resilient surface like a mouse pad.) This has the effect of energizing the remedy. You can succuss it ten times or so between sips.

## Hypersensitives Need a Milder Dose

Occasionally we come across someone who is sensitive to everything—to medications, vitamins, and all kinds of chemicals and fumes—and to every homeopathic remedy you give them. These people are called "hypersensitives" and you know who you are!

For hypersensitives, use a 6c potency, much milder than the 30c standard potency for self care. Health food stores may not have this mild potency. (Some stores carry the 12c potency, which may also work for hypersensitives.)

You can order a First Aid Emergency Kit from Natural Health Supply (see page 202) in a 6c strength. Maybe 5% to 10% of my clients need this hypersensitive dose, and maybe 5% to 10% need a much stronger dose like a 100c or even 200c.

## Vegan? Lactose Intolerant? Diabetic? Avoiding Sugar?

Homeopathic remedy pellets (like the hard round pellets in the blue tube) are usually made from sucrose while the soft tablets (like Hylands, cell salts) are made from lactose. The amount of either is insignificant, especially if you use the tiny pellets from Natural Health Supply.

I have never had a lactose intolerant or diabetic client react to the sugar in a remedy. However, to be on the safe side, you can dissolve the pellets in water, as described on the previous page, and take just a small sip as a dose.

If you're totally opposed to milk products for religious or philosophical reasons, you should know that even the pellets contain a tiny percentage of lactose to hold the sucrose together. They are still a better option for you than the soft flat tablets, which are pure lactose.

Also a few, very few remedies are made from animal substances. Apis, Calcarea carbonica, Cantharis, Lachesis and Sepia are the only animal-based remedies out of the 100 most commonly-used ones. In the case of Lachesis and Sepia, the remedy can be made without killing the animal. In the case of Apis, Calc. carb. and Cantharis, one bee or bug or oyster shell can be diluted to make millions of doses.

## Giving the Remedies to a Baby

These remedies have been used safely for 200 years now for millions of people—including babies. The FDA allows their use for babies and small children. Just be careful that your baby doesn't choke on a remedy pellet. Here's how to avoid that:

- If you get the kit I recommend, the pellets are tiny, like a grain of sand, and you can safely tuck one inside your baby's mouth.
- If you get a "blue tube" from the health food store, the pellets are bigger, the size of a pea, so you'll need to crush them into a powder and put a bit into your baby's mouth.
- You can dissolve the powder in a little water and dab it onto your baby's lips, or even onto the temples—the remedy will absorb

through the delicate skin—and you may feel more comfortable applying the remedy externally, especially if you're new to these remedies (and/or new to being a parent). You'll feel more comfortable with these remedies as you become more experienced and discover how safe they are.

**"Help! My child swallowed the whole tube!"** Not a problem. If it was your child's remedy, she might have a brief aggravation (worsening). If the remedy wasn't her well-matched remedy, her system won't react.

### Safety First

Sometimes people get so passionate about natural healing, they avoid doctors and hospitals at all costs. But we need doctors and hospitals. There are some things that just can't be treated at home. Please use common sense and don't go overboard.

In an emergency situation where you would have called 9-1-1, gone to the emergency room, or called your doctor before you learned about natural healing—**still do that.** Remember the guidelines on page 45.

---

#### A NURSE WHO WOULDN'T GO TO THE HOSPITAL

A nurse who was studying homeopathy with me called me for a remedy suggestion, saying, "I know my little boy has appendicitis but I don't want to take him to the hospital because I'm afraid they will give him antibiotics and that will mess up his system."

I said, "Take him to the hospital! The antibiotics could save his life! We can do something about the antibiotics later!" I refrained from saying, "Are you crazy?" Please don't be too fanatical about natural remedies.

---

## Giving Remedies Before Surgery

"I want to give the pre-surgery remedies but my instructions say NPO, Nothing By Mouth."

What the instructions really mean is not to swallow anything before the operation which you might vomit up and then breathe into your lungs — big trouble.

The remedies dissolve in the mouth **so you won't be swallowing anything.** That means it's fine to take them before surgery.

If you want to follow your pre-surgery instructions literally, though, you can dissolve each remedy in a little water and dab it onto your lips, temples, inside of your wrists — your body's healing energy will still "get the message."

Because it's hard to give remedies in the hospital, it's best to take them before you leave for the hospital.

Some day, conventional doctors and hospitals may come to know what a wonderful, helpful, and safe support these remedies are — and perhaps someday the remedies will be part of the before-and-after surgery protocol in every hospital.

In the meantime, we need to respect their restrictions, which are based on a concern for your safety and the need to protect people against substances that they're not familiar with.

## Giving the Remedies After Surgery

You'll most likely need to wait until the patient comes home because the staff will not allow you to give anything they are not familiar with.

One way to get around this: dissolve the remedies in a small bottle of water and label it "holy water." Is it really holy water? Yes, if you believe it is. It is healing water, and healing is a sacred act. Nurses are trained to respect your religious beliefs and will treat your "holy water" with respect.

**Tooth Extractions:** follow the same instructions.

# HOW DO THE REMEDIES WORK?

Here's where cutting-edge developments in mainstream medicine meet the 200-year-old science of homeopathy. The hot news in conventional medicine now is *nanoparticles*— particles so tiny, they are only one atom or molecule wide along one edge. Nanoparticles change the behavior of *other* particles in a solution so dramatically that they're now being used to deliver medications like chemotherapy drugs. The amount of the drug needed is greatly reduced, thereby reducing side effects for the patient and costs for the health care system.

Apparently homeopathic medicines work on the same principle. They are made by taking a small amount of the source material (usually an herb, sometimes a mineral or animal product), repeatedly diluting it in distilled water, and giving it a series of vigorous succussions (whacks) against a resilient surface. Dilution alone does not create medicinally-active remedies. (In fact dilution alone makes them weaker, just as you would expect.)

Rather, the succussions at each step of dilution release tiny fragments of glass (silica), which are then turned into nanoparticles along with the remedy substance. Interestingly, silica nanoparticles have been found in conventional medicine to form one of the best carriers for other substances!

What goes on in a homeopathic remedy solution has been a mystery up until now, because we had no instruments powerful enough to detect the presence of nanoparticles. But recently scientists at the Indian Institute of Technology in Bombay detected the presence of nanoparticles of the original starting substance, in homeopathic remedies so dilute that they could not possibly contain even a molecule of the substance according to the chemistry we studied in high school. These medicinally active nanoparticles, along with nanoparticles of silica from the glass container, form a highly effective delivery system. We can no longer say about a homeopathic remedy, "There's nothing in it."

There must be more to it than nanoparticles, though. In conventional medicine, nanoparticles deliver a drug like a chemotherapy drug more effectively, so that less is needed to get the same effect. In homeopathy, a substance that has no healing effect (or may even have a toxic effect) becomes a medicine in nanoparticle form. How is this possible?

The medicinal substance in a homeopathic remedy does more than act like a drug. It seems to convey information, like an energetic template. It appears to communicate with the body's healing energy, reminding the body of its natural healthy state. Imagine a tree falls through the roof of your garage and you need to repair it. You need lumber, shingles and other building supplies, true. These are like the nutritional supplements needed to heal chronic disease. But you also need the architect's drawings so that you know where all the lumber and shingles go. That appears to be what the homeopathic remedy does.

I like to think of the tiny homeopathic pellets as computer chips, each storing a tremendous amount of information. Apparently in the fast-evolving world of computer technology, storage devices are being developed which contain only a dozen molecules — in other words, the size of nanoparticles. Homeopathic remedy particles may also act as storage devices for healing information. Is it a coincidence that silicon is the basis for information storage in computers, while silica (a silicon compound) seems to provide the most effective nanoparticles for drug delivery? Neither a chemist nor a physicist, I am looking forward to someone else shedding light on this question.

Another aspect of homeopathy's mechanism of action is the structured or coherent water in a remedy solution. Ordinary water has water molecules bumping into each other like little bumper cars. In some situations, though, these molecules start to attract each other and form complex patterns in the water—way too small to be seen by the naked eye, but detectable with an electron microscope. The water molecules aren't rigidly bound together as they would be in an ice crystal, but they are interacting in a crystal-like structured pattern. This highly organized water seems to deliver dissolved substances much more effectively, as described in Gannon and Lo's *Double Helix Water.*

So how do these explanations fit together? The science is still evolving. Stay tuned because exciting new research is coming out all the time to explain how homeopathy works.

What happens once the remedy is in your body is still unknown. That just means the technology does not yet exist to detect its action. I'm reminded of the case of acupuncture, which was developed five thousand years ago when Chinese healers—who must have been extremely sensitive to energy fields—detected the presence of lines or *meridians* of energy flow which were more intense at certain vortex points (these became the acupuncture points). Within the past few years, instruments were developed which could scan the electromagnetic field of the body, and lo and behold, they revealed the presence of concentrated areas of more intense energy corresponding to the meridians and acupuncture points of Chinese medicine. Acupuncture worked long before Western science could "prove" it, and the same is likely to be true of homeopathy.

### How Come I've Never Heard of Homeopathy?

The remedies are not patentable; they are in the public domain. A tube of a homeopathic remedy that costs $7.95 in a health food store can last you for years.

As a result, there are no extra funds generated to publicize homeopathy. Homeopathic drug manufacturers can't afford TV commercials, ads in medical journals, or sales reps visiting doctors' offices. Most people find out about it through word of mouth from satisfied users. Please tell your friends!

## What to Say to a Skeptic

My father the doctor helped me a lot in writing this book—by arguing with just about everything in it. "Where are the research studies?" he would say. "Show me the double-blind, randomized, placebo-controlled studies on this stuff and then I'll try it." So here is my answer to my own personal skeptic.

Here's the deal, dad.

Nobody's giving us money to research these remedies. Well, actually, the NIH has given teeny-weeny amounts of money to study homeopathic medicines for chronic illnesses, and the results were positive, clearly better than placebo. But this book is about home care and there's no research money for natural home care.

This book is about trying things that are safe, especially in situations where conventional medicine has little to offer. It's about listening to your body, noticing what works, trusting your own experience. It's about natural medicines that have 200 years of clinical experience to back up their safety and effectiveness.

"Let's take the case of smoking," I said—a topic dear to my father's heart. As a vascular surgeon (specializing in blood vessel surgery) he was a pioneer in recommending natural lifestyles. He would require his patients to stop smoking, start exercising, and change to a low-fat diet, decades before these interventions became popular.

And he set a good example for his patients. He stopped smoking (he only smoked a pipe—ah, the aroma!—but he learned it could cause tongue and lip cancer). He started running marathons. He would get up at 4:30 in the morning so he could complete his marathon training and still get to the hospital by 7 am. If his patients told him they didn't have time to exercise, he brushed off the excuse. "If I have time, you have time," he would tell them.

"So dad, what if back in the 1960s, one of your colleagues told you he had noticed that his clients who stopped smoking had better circulation—based on their reports of fewer leg cramps, less shortness of breath while walking uphill, and no more cold hands and feet. Would you have started recommending right away that your patients stop smoking, knowing that they would get other benefits even if they weren't able to avoid surgery?

"Or would you refuse to recommend it until the research studies were completed, which could take 10 years? And what if no one would pay for the studies, since no industry would benefit from them? Would you go ahead and urge your patients to stop smoking anyway?"

"Sure," dad says. "Right away. No need to wait for the research."

"So it's the same with my stuff," I said. "It's harmless. It's likely to bring about other health benefits. There's no money for research studies. There are a lot of people telling us that it works for them. Like a little melt-in-your-mouth tablet that might help with those stomach cramps of yours."

"Okay," my 85-year-old surgeon-father says. "Let's try some of that."

And here's more I could add for other skeptics—yours, perhaps.

I see a lot of contradictory arguments against homeopathy: that there's nothing in it, and that it's dangerous.

And a lot of critics say it's "unproven," which is not true—there is extensive research supporting it—but in any case, remember that "unproven" does not mean "proven not to work." It means "not tested yet," due to lack of funds.

It's also said to work by the placebo effect, but that can't be true because it works on infants, animals, even on plants. Anyone who has given a remedy to a baby screaming with teething pain, and watched the child stop crying instantaneously, knows that it cannot possibly be the placebo effect. Even a narcotic couldn't work that fast.

Nor can the effect be based on a pleasant experience with a professional homeopath, as some claim. (This is my father's theory. "You're a nice person and people like talking to you. That's why they feel better.") No matter how supportive the experience, no matter how much the client enjoys feeling truly heard, the remedy will not work if it is not a good match.

The best proof of homeopathy's effectiveness is personal experience. Try the remedies in this book. Sometimes homeopathy does not work well for a particular person, but if you keep trying it on several people, you *will* see it work.

There *is* plenty of research, though most of it has been conducted overseas where homeopathy is an accepted part of the health care system. Dana Ullman has done such a thorough job of keeping track of this research and describing it, that I'll simply refer you to his Huffington Post blogs and to his website, **www.homeopathic.com**. His e-book, *Homeopathic Family Medicine*, is worth getting because it documents the research for dozens of common complaints while providing more extensive remedy recommendations than I can give here. It references more than 200 clinical studies that have been published in peer-reviewed medical journals, listed in the chapter for each condition.

A dramatic and compelling book about the science behind homeopathy is Dr. Amy Lansky's *Impossible Cure*. Lansky was a NASA computer scientist whose autistic son was cured with homeopathy (that's why it's called *Impossible Cure*, because conventional medicine considers autism incurable). She was so impressed that she left NASA to become a professional homeopath. Her book interweaves a report on the research documenting homeopathy with the compelling story of her son, who has now graduated from college. (It was written before the new research on nanoparticles came out, though.)

The Swiss government has spent five years thoroughly examining the safety, effectiveness, and cost-effectiveness of homeopathy (with typical Swiss neutrality) and has decided to keep covering it in their national health insurance. The report itself is quite dry, but you don't need to read it because Dana Ullman has done an excellent job of summarizing it in his Huffington Post blog.

### How Come My Doctor Says It's Unproven?

Chances are your doctor is not familiar with the research on homeopathy, which is understandable, since most of the research has been done overseas and is not taught in American medical schools.

Homeopathic drug manufacturers cannot afford to fund research the way American drug companies do. The US government has funded a few studies which have demonstrated the effectiveness of homeopathy and have published in peer-reviewed journals (for example, on homeopathy for childhood diarrhea and for mild traumatic brain injury).

To reassure your doctor, try telling her or him that homeopathy is an accepted part of the national health care system in many countries around the world and that FDA regulations in this country are comparable to those for drugs. In other words, the FDA oversees it as a system of medicine comparable to mainstream medicine, quite differently from how the FDA regulates vitamins and herbs.

Doctors don't have time to study natural healing. They can't keep up with the information in their own specialty. Please be respectful and appreciative of all that doctors *do* know, and share your success stories about your natural medicine cabinet. Doctors will become more comfortable with natural healing the more they hear about their patients using it.

### Why Is Wikipedia So Negative about Homeopathy?

The editorial board at Wikipedia (which is not as neutral as they would like us to believe) has been suppressing attempts by homeopaths to post accurate information. Anything positive posted about homeopathy is immediately deleted, including references to research articles refuting the negative statements in the Wikipedia article. Homeopaths apparently are not allowed to post to the article because they have a conflict of interest, even though medical doctors can post information about conventional medicine.

# WIIAT DOES THE
# LABEL MEAN?

Get out your magnifying glass and let's take a look at the label on a homeopathic medicine. It has:

**The full Latin name of the medicine.** Most homeopathic medicines are made from plants, and most of the rest from minerals. Either way, you get long Latin words which are often hard to pronounce, so in this book I've used nicknames such as Nat. mur. for Natrum muriaticum or Rhus. tox. for Rhus toxicodendron.

**A number followed by a letter C or X.** The higher the number, the stronger the medicine. The goal is not to use the *strongest* one you can find, but the one that *suits you the best*. X refers to the Roman numeral for 10 (as in "decimal") and is usually only used for cell salts (page 168).

**A condition that the medicine will treat.** The condition on the label is probably not the one you're trying to treat. Each homeopathic medicine can treat many different conditions but only one will fit on the label. Each condition may respond to multiple remedies and each remedy can treat multiple conditions, because you're trying to match the remedy to your *individual, unique* symptoms like getting fitted for a custom-tailored suit. It's fun, like a challenging puzzle, and the prize is that your symptoms go away!

**Directions for use.** There is no way to anticipate all the different conditions the medicine might be used for, so the manufacturer gives a conservative recommendation, in other words one that is so mild it's unlikely anyone will have an aggravation (temporary worsening of symptoms). But taking the remedy twice a day, as recommended, is often not sufficient. So then you might think the remedy doesn't work. I try to give more flexible guidelines on pages 204–208.

**An expiration date.** This is a legal technicality. Homeopathic medicines do not expire if they are in a tightly-capped container, unless they are exposed to high heat. Don't leave them in the glove compartment of your car on a hot day. Once opened, they'll be fine unless you leave the cover off in a steamy bathroom or a medicine cabinet with strong-smelling salves.

If you open a tube and the pellets are not melted and stuck together, they should be fine no matter what the expiration date says.

---

### A Husband with Hot Flashes?

One of my clients asked me to help her husband, who had a sore throat. I talked to him on the phone and determined that he most likely needed Lachesis, a medicine for left-sided sore throats. I told him he could get it at Cambridge Naturals, which was much closer than picking it up at my office.

His wife called me shortly thereafter. He had come back in disgust because the label said it was for hot flashes. I explained that just as each *condition* could be addressed by many different *medicines* (hence my lengthy questioning about his sore throat), so too each *medicine* can help with many different *conditions*. And yes, I really did mean Lachesis for his sore throat.

## What If I'm Pregnant or Nursing?

If you read the fine print on the label, you'll find something like this: "If pregnant or breastfeeding, ask a health professional before use."

I wish it said, "Ask a professional homeopath before use," because if you ask your doctor, chances are he/she won't know anything about it because it wasn't covered in medical school. Doctors take on legal liability if anything goes wrong with something they have approved. So doctors understandably err on the side of caution with pregnant patients.

Here's the lowdown. On the one hand, it's safe to use homeopathic medicines while pregnant. (We'll deal with breastfeeding separately—it's a bit more complicated.) How do we know? 200 years of experience, millions of women who've done it, thousands of professionals who have monitored them. Apparently in the heyday of homeopathy, a hundred or more years ago in this country, the labor and delivery nurses preferred the homeopathic hospitals to the allopathic hospitals (the ones using what we now consider conventional medicine). They found that women using homeopathy during pregnancy had shorter and easier deliveries, with less pain and fewer complications.

If I were pregnant, I would use homeopathy, and I would give it to a pregnant friend or sister, without a moment's hesitation. But if you are pregnant, you need to make your own decision. Here's why.

When a woman is pregnant, her baby is profoundly affected by her state of mind. For more on this, see Rita Kluny's wonderful book *Your Baby Remembers: Parenting with a Deep Heart from the Start*. It cites research not readily available on how unborn babies do indeed remember their mother's emotional state. (The book provides techniques for parents and grandparents to provide emotional healing through loving touch. Highly recommended.)

If a woman is new to homeopathy and her family is doubtful, her ob/gyn even more so, it can create anxiety which could outweigh the benefits of the remedy.

Homeopathy could work well, though, for a couple from India whose family on both sides have used homeopathy for generations, and who has found an Indian ob/gyn here in the US who is experienced with homeopathy. Or for a crunchy granola type, if she and her partner have used herbs for years, many of their friends have used homeopathy for pregnancy, and they're working with a midwife trained in homeopathy. These pregnant women will receive support, not anxiety, from their families and community for using homeopathy.

So please consider your situation. If you are new to homeopathy, pregnancy is not the best time to start experimenting. The most important thing when you're pregnant is to send your baby love, not anxiety. (If you notice yourself getting anxious, take some deep breaths, focus on your heart, and send love from your heart to your baby's.)

As for nursing, homeopathy for the mother is generally considered safe for the baby. Some homeopaths have found that medicines taken by the mother will go through the breast milk to the baby. In fact, this method can be used as a way of administering a medicine to a baby, if mother and baby need the same medicine.)

But what if the baby doesn't need the medicine? It's unlikely to affect the baby, for the same reason that a baby can swallow a whole tube of the medicine without any effect. The body doesn't respond if it doesn't need the remedy, like when a tuning fork is struck: a tuning fork at the same pitch will vibrate while a tuning fork at a different pitch will not respond.

To be on the safe side, though, many homeopaths recommend that a nursing mother take her daily dose of a medicine after the breastfeeding when she's likely to have the longest stretch of time before the next one. We don't really have a way to test whether this matters. I am not aware of any record in the literature of a baby reacting to a medicine taken by a breastfeeding mother.

Speaking of testing, you may wonder why the medicines have these warning labels at all. That's because the FDA requires them on *all* medications unless they have gone through extensive testing on pregnant and breastfeeding women. Think about it. If you were pregnant, would you sign up to be part of a research study on an unknown medicine? Right. That's why we don't have the research studies.

# FOR MORE INFORMATION

If you'd like to really get how homeopathy works, I would use the **Mastering Natural Remedies** series of video seminars, featuring internationally distinguished author and lecturer Miranda Castro. Filmed when Miranda was teaching in Boston, it includes her answers to practical questions from participants just like you. Miranda's seminars are vivid, entertaining, and full of stories that help you remember the remedies and how to use them. If you like the stories in this book, you'll love Miranda's videos. She's funny, she's British, she's a great teacher.

To purchase them in DVD form: **www.MirandaCastro.com**.

To stream the videos: **www.YourNaturalMedicineCabinet.com**.

∾ **Homeopathy 101** covers basic first aid, accidents, injuries, preparing for surgery—much more detail, more conditions and more remedies than in this book.

∾ **StressBusters** covers emotional traumas and remedies for all kinds of fears and anxieties. It's essential for a deeper understanding because it explains how homeopaths think about causation—that chronic illnesses can be caused by emotional trauma (grief, fright, humiliation, abuse) or mental strain (too much study or computer work) as well as physical factors like a head injury or mercury toxicity.

∾ **The Twelve Fabulous Cell Salts** covers these universally useful, really safe remedies. (This one only from **www.MirandaCastro.com**.)

Just a couple more recommendations, available from Homeopathic Educational Services, **www.Homeopathic.com.** This is the best source because they have so many resources and so much free information about homeopathy.

᭦ *Everybody's Guide to Homeopathic Medicines* by Cummings and Ullman covers many more conditions than we cover here, and gives more remedy options for the conditions in this book. For each condition it tells you the warning signs that you should call your doctor, head for the hospital, or even call 9-1-1.

᭦ *A Homeopathic Guide to Stress* by Miranda Castro

᭦ *Homeopathic Medicines for Children and Infants* by Dana Ullman (essential if you have kids)

᭦ *Whole Woman Homeopathy* by Judyth Reichenberg-Ullman

᭦ *Beauty in Bloom* by Eileen Naumann (about menopause)

᭦ *Musculoskeletal Healing with Homeopathy* by Asa Hershoff (covers headaches, sciatica, arthritis, back pain, and more).

**Books that explain homeopathy**

᭦ *Impossible Cure* by Dr. Amy Lansky (described on page 217 in the section about research) is my favorite introductory book to explain homeopathy.

᭦ *Prozac-Free, Ritalin-Free Kids* and *Rage-Free Kids* by Robert Ullman and Judyth Reichenberg-Ullman explain the value of homeopathic treatment for psychological and behavioral issues.

᭦ *Emotional Healing with Homeopathy* by Peter Chappell.

᭦ *Nature and Human Personality* by Catherine Coulter (the distinguished homeopath, not the author of popular fiction). This just might be the most entertaining introduction because it describes the personality types of the most common remedies. You'll recognize your spouse, your boss, your mom . . . and you'll know what remedies often work for them, based on their personality traits. Fun!

᭦ *The Homeopathic Revolution* by Dana Ullman is about all the famous people in history who have used homeopathy, whether pop stars, popes or presidents. More fun!

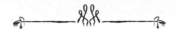

## PART FIVE

# YOUR SUPPORT SYSTEM

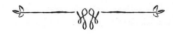

Good information about natural healing is not enough.
You need an inner attitude of strength and self-confidence,
a kind of inner knowing. Some people gain the most confidence
by studying the research, others by feedback via lab tests,
still others by learning to self-test with applied
kinesiology (muscle testing).

From years of teaching, I've found that people master new material
best when they process it in all three "channels": reading and
writing about it, hearing about it and explaining it to others,
and experiencing it for themselves. Find buddies so that you
can talk about your new experiences and learn together.

You also need a positive environment, and that means
people around you who respect your interest in natural healing:
your friends, family, and physicians. If you have a chronic illness,
you'll need to find a health care practitioner specializing in natural
treatment methods which are beyond the scope of this book.

In this section you'll find out how to test yourself,
how to find supportive friends and practitioners,
and how to locate a natural health care professional.

# LEARN TO CHECK
# FOR YOURSELF

You can gain confidence in natural healing, depending on your inclination, by studying the latest research . . . by getting yourself tested . . . and by learning how to test yourself. Here are some quick and easy ways.

### What's the Latest Research?

If you're a science wonk, check out **www.CamResearch.net**. Also try **www. GreenMedInfo.com**, and the Research tab at **www.NutraSpace.com**.

For the latest research on homeopathy, join the National Center for Homeopathy (**www.NationalCenterforHomeopathy.org**). Lots of exciting new developments here, both in the physics of how remedies work and in the specific conditions they're good for . . . even for cancer, according to research at MD Anderson, one of the world's leading cancer institutes.

### Get Yourself Tested

**Vitamin D:** most people are surprisingly low, compared to the Vitamin D Council's recommended blood levels of 50 to 80. If your insurance does not cover vitamin D testing, you can get a discount on a home test on their website, **www.VitaminDCouncil.org**. You may need to diplomatically remind your doctor how important vitamin D is for bone strength, a healthy immune system, even for seasonal affective disorder. Also remind your doctor that it has to be the 25(OH)D test.

**Acid/alkaline balance:** This has a huge impact on a wide variety of health conditions. You want your body to be slightly alkaline, but a lot of factors in our American lifestyle tend to be acidifying: sugar, alcohol, meat, stress. Sound familiar? You can test your body's pH with little urine dip-strips, available at drug stores and health food stores. If you're acidic, start your day with the juice of half a lemon in a glass of water. Lemons have an alkalinizing effect on the body even though they taste acidic. Or use the cell salt Nat. phos. (see page 176), and eat lots of green vegetables. More info on acid/alkaline balance easily available online and in health food stores, for example in Felicia Kliment's *The Acid-Alkaline Balance Diet*.

**Other self-tests** (using blood, saliva, or stool samples which you collect yourself at home and send in to a lab) can reveal really important things about your body, from parasites (yes, civilized people get them) to adrenal function. You'll need a naturopath or holistic doctor to interpret the results and guide you on supplementation, but it's good to know they're available to help you take charge of your health. For example, see *Life Changers: Ten Painless High-Tech Home Medical Tests* by Dr. Edward J. Conley.

**Blood pressure:** If you have high blood pressure, get a blood pressure cuff and test yourself regularly at home. This will overcome the "white coat effect" (people get nervous at the doctor's office and their blood pressure tends to be higher than normal).

**Otoscope:** If you have a child who gets ear infections a lot, get an otoscope (the instrument used to look into a child's ear). Start checking when your child is healthy, so you know what a healthy eardrum looks like for comparison, and search YouTube for video instructions.

## Tuning In to Your Body

You can learn to test yourself by using applied kinesiology (muscle testing) to tune in to your body's wisdom. Sounds woo-woo, it's not. Lots of people do this, including all the health care practitioners in my office.

One simple way to do it: form a circle by touching the tip of your forefinger to the tip of your thumb. Insert the forefinger and thumb of your other hand into the circle. They will be straight and flat against each other like pincers. Try to open them gently so that they break the circle formed by the other two fingers. You'll have to play around with this a bit to see how hard to try to pry them apart.

Experiment by placing in front of you a healthy food or supplement that you are sure is good for you, and feel how strong that "finger circle" is when you look at the food.

Now place some items in front of you that are likely to be harmful for your body. (We keep some conventional household cleaning agents in the office just for this purpose.) Try opening your "finger circle" with your "pincer fingers" and see how weak you feel and how easy it is to break the circle.

Of course, if you press hard enough with your "pincer fingers," you can always break the circle formed by your other fingers, but then you won't learn anything. Play around with it until you can feel the difference.

This is much simpler than it sounds. It's hard to describe, easy to do. There's a demo on YouTube: look for "Muscle Testing" uploaded by FitLife.tv. (It's one of the few videos that show *self*-testing, although there are many YouTube videos that show how someone else can do it for you.) Try it, give it a couple of weeks, see if it works for you as an indicator.

Muscle testing yourself may not be as accurate as having a professional do it for you (because it's hard to be neutral when testing yourself). A health care professional experienced in using applied kinesiology can use it to diagnose health conditions that are hard to detect with conventional testing.

But for ordinary decisions, like whether a food will support your health or not, muscle testing yourself can help you refine your choices.

# FIND YOUR
# KINDRED SPIRITS

Do you feel like you are the only one among your family and friends who is into this natural lifestyle stuff? You are not alone—you are part of a groundswell of change, a transformation that's happening in our society. It's just that at this point, pioneers like you are scattered.

You need to find your kindred spirits. For years I've heard moms in my practice say, "I'm the *only* mother I know who is trying to keep her kids off sugar and away from the computer, feed them healthy food, get them outside to play. . ." and for years I've wished I could get these moms together, but they lived too far apart. Now Holistic Moms is creating this kind of community. It's a great way to share information, true—but more importantly, it creates emotional support for all of you who feel like you're swimming upstream in this heavily commercialized culture. **www.HolisticMoms.org** is both an online community and in some locales, a meet-up group.

You might also find a Pathways to Wellness Gathering Group. These educational meetings are based on an excellent and informative magazine, *Pathways to Wellness*. It's put out by a group of chiropractors and the meetings are often held in a chiropractic practice. See **www. PathwaysToFamilyWellness.org** for a location near you where you can pick up this great magazine and meet some likeminded folks.

Can't find either one nearby? Try **www.Meetup.com**. Put in your zip code, or that of the nearest large city, and try keywords like "holistic" or "natural healing," and you'll meet interesting people enthusiastic about sharing their knowledge and experience.

If you can't find a meetup, it's easy to start one. You'll get support and great suggestions from like-minded people.

And remember, some day the same people who are now poking fun at your healthy lifestyle may be turning to you for advice. I've seen it happen many times: the fringe member of a family or neighborhood or PTA becomes the go-to person when others run into health problems that conventional medicine can't fix.

# THE "INTERNET DOCTOR"

The internet is both a blessing and a curse in giving you information about potential disease conditions. I mostly find that my clients who research possible diseases on the internet end up scaring themselves unnecessarily.

The "internet doctor" is great, though, if you have a new strange symptom in the middle of the night and you're trying to figure out what it might be and how urgently to address it. Here are three such sites, and it would be wise to check all three:

- **HealthWise:** www.Health.msn.com/health-topics. This is my favorite because it seems to have the most intelligent "decision tree," a good list of home care recommendations, and a list of new symptoms that might arise, indicating the need for urgent action.
- **The Mayo Clinic:** www.MayoClinic.com/health/symptom-checker
- **Harvard Medical School**'s site: www.SymptomChecker.about.com.

If your symptoms point to either a minor, common condition or a rare fatal one, assume it's the minor one until you can get to a doctor — don't worry yourself sick.

And by the way, the internet is an unusually poor source of information about homeopathy. What's on the net tends to be outdated. My clients who look up their homeopathic medicine on the internet find Victorian-era disease descriptions plus some outlandish "delusions," because this material pre-dates a modern understanding of psychology.

I had one client who refused to take what I gave her because the internet said it was for "delusions of grandeur" (*not!*) and she was offended at the description.

The internet does have useful resources about homeopathy in general, especially the exciting field of new research in homeopathy — research that's documenting how it works and its effectiveness in diseases like cancer. But the information about specific remedies is worse than useless when trying to understand your own case. Even worse are the simplistic online homoopathic software sites (you tell it your symptoms, it tells you your remedy). My clients have been totally misdirected by these sites.

If you want to find a remedy for a condition not covered by this book, you'll get better results with one of the books on page 224.

# PARTNER WITH YOUR PRIMARY CARE DOCTOR

When treating your children, and especially babies, you want to be extra sure that you are doing it safely. The guidelines in this book for what's safe to treat at home are only general guidelines for basically healthy people.

For example, if your child's fever starts to rise, you'll want to know how high the fever can go before you really do need to give a conventional medicine. There's no hard and fast rule—it depends on several factors including your child's overall demeanor, other symptoms, and medical history.

You need to work with your doctor, so if you want to use natural remedies for home care, it's best to find a doctor who is supportive. If they are not, they will automatically tell you to bring in anyone who is sick. But going to a doctor's office (or even worse, an emergency room) can expose you to further contagion. Plus you can become overmedicalized, getting tests and drugs you do not need.

If your doctor is overly skeptical or sarcastic, if your doctor makes fun of your efforts or makes you feel stupid, it is time to find another doctor. Most doctors, though, are simply skeptical of something they are unfamiliar with.

While doctors in many other countries around the world are trained in natural medicines or refer patients to their colleagues who are, American medical schools have only recently begun including some reference to natural healing. And the American Medical Association has only recently recommended that doctors educate themselves about alternative practices.

Once you get good results with natural healing, try telling your doctor. The more doctors hear about this from their patients, the more comfortable they'll be with these modalities.

Your doctor may say these remedies are "unproven." But these natural medicinals often *do* have research behind them, research published overseas which your doctor is not familiar with. Homeopathic medicines have a 200-year track record of safe and effective use. Herbal medicines would not have survived for hundreds and thousands of years if they were not safe.

You may not need to search for an open-minded MD to act as your Primary Care Physician (PCP). If you are lucky, you can get a *real* nature-doctor—called a naturopath.

**Naturopaths** are health care professionals who go through years of training comparable to medical school, except they learn how to use natural remedies, herbs, vitamins, and healthy food instead of drugs. In about 15 to 20 states, naturopaths can act as primary care physicians.

Check **www.naturopathic.org**, click on About Naturopathic Medicine, then Licensure to see if they are licensed in your state. If so, you can check the directory listing for your state on the same website. If not, you can still have a family naturopath (which I highly recommend). You'll just have to pay out of pocket and your naturopath will not be able to order medical tests or write prescriptions as they can in "licensed" states. People who pay out of pocket for natural health care tend to save money anyway, because they get sick less often and have fewer co-pays.

Here are some other approaches to finding an open-minded PCP.

You may find that **nurse practitioners** are more open-minded about natural methods than doctors are, because nurses' training tends to be more holistic. In many states nurse practitioners can act as primary care providers. You may also find that women and younger doctors, in general, are more open-minded (although I also hear of grandmotherly practitioners who fondly remember the home remedies of their youth).

Here's what you *don't* need: a physician listed as a *practitioner* of holistic medicine, for example on the American Holistic Medical Association website (**www.HolisticMedicine.org**).

These people (also known as functional medicine doctors) are real specialists in treating chronic diseases with supplements, and they often don't take insurance. They rarely act as primary care physicians because they are in such demand. They're likely to be too busy to respond to emergencies.

You are not asking your PCP to be the *expert* in natural remedies, you just want a doctor who will support you in *your* efforts. To find one, you could ask at your local health food store. The folks there are likely to know who's in town and who's good.

Or ask a trusted acupuncturist, chiropractor, homeopath, naturopath, massage therapist, or other holistic professional if they have a favorite PCP. You could also try the members of your local Holistic Moms group (see page 230). Their website, **www.HolisticMoms.org,** is a great way for like-minded parents to share info like this.

# FIND A HOLISTIC
# HEALTH CARE PROFESSIONAL

This book is meant to support you in treating *acute* (current) conditions. You'll need professional help for *chronic* (longterm) conditions. Your best options are a physician who specializes in functional medicine, a naturopathic doctor, or a professional homeopath. How to choose?

A physician specializing in functional medicine is a fully trained and licensed conventional doctor who prefers to work with supplements rather than drugs. Advantages include their knowledge of conventional medicine and their ability to monitor any necessary prescription medications. On the other hand, these doctors are in great demand. Your community may not have any, or they may not be taking new patients. They probably won't take insurance because they spend much more time with patients than insurance will cover. They usually prescribe a lot of supplements, which are likely to be expensive and not covered by insurance. Their services are totally worth it if you can possibly afford them. You will most probably save a lifetime of co-pays and prescription drug expenses.

If you have a serious, potentially life-threatening illness, especially one for which you are already on medication, I would recommend going to such a physician even if it involves traveling to another city and paying out of pocket. Bottom line: these physicians may not be easy to find, but they are well worth seeking out.

Another good reason to seek out a functional medicine doctor is simply the confidence and credibility factor. You may have a family member who will *only* see an MD, even though a naturopathic doctor or professional homeopath may be just as capable of helping him.

Naturopathic doctors may provide the best of both worlds. You want to be sure that they have graduated from one of the five accredited schools of naturopathy in the US and Canada (Bastyr, Boucher Institute, Canadian College of Naturopathic Medicine, National College, the National University of Health Sciences, Southwest College, or the University of Bridgeport). These doctors have been through a curriculum similar to medical school, except that they learn about supplements, herbs, and other holistic modalities instead of drugs. Beware of people calling themselves naturopaths who received their training online, which in no way compares to four years of full-time school followed by internships in hospitals and doctors' offices. (I'll make an exception for oldtimey nature-doctors who've been in practice since before these accredited schools even existed. You'll find them by word of mouth.)

In some states naturopathic doctors are even licensed to practice as primary care doctors. If this were true in my state, I would definitely use a naturopath as my PCP. The differences between a functional medicine doctor and a naturopathic doctor are minimal. The former knows more about conventional medicine, the latter knows more about natural healing modalities like acupuncture, chiropractic and detoxification, and both know a lot about nutrition, vitamins and herbs. So the difference may not matter in your case. You might choose based on insurance coverage, proximity, and word of mouth.

How about a professional homeopath? Homeopathy shines when there is a mind-body component to the chronic condition. Here are a couple of ways you can tell:

- if your condition is worse when you are under stress or experiencing a strong emotion such as anger or grief
- or if your condition started at the same time you were going through a major stress.

Homeopaths call this concept the "Never Well Since," as in "I've never been the same since . . . " (my husband left me, or I lost all my money in the dotcom crash, or my son was killed in a car accident, or I had to work for an abusive and humiliating boss . . .).

Homeopathy is also based on the concept of healing the whole person. It has the remarkable ability to reach back in time and heal a past stress or trauma. I can't explain how, but I have seen it happen many times in my practice. People come in ostensibly for a physical condition and then they find that their whole mood and energy level and self-image are so much improved that they hardly notice that their physical problem went away too.

The qualifications for being a homeopath are trickier than for naturopathy or functional medicine, so please bear with me while I explain a bit more about how to find a homeopath. And the bottom line is this: all three types of practitioners (functional medicine doctor, naturopath, homeopath) are rare enough that you might not have a choice, unless you live in a bicoastal urban area. If there is even one practitioner in your community doing any of these three types of healing, and if that person has a good reputation, I would go see him or her.

A good resource for finding all different kinds of holistic practitioners is Jill's List, at **www.JillsList.com**, because they check to make sure that all practitioners on their site are licensed or nationally certified. This is really important in the current state of affairs, which is a bit of a Wild West in terms of credentialing. Many holistic professions are not regulated by the government, so that anyone can hang out a shingle after a modicum of training.

## How to Find a Professional Homeopath

A professional homeopath is someone who uses homeopathy as their only (or primary) modality, not someone who uses it for minor symptom relief while addressing your health condition with another practice like acupuncture or chiropractic.

A professional homeopath may or may not have a license in another health care modality (except in a couple of states, where they are *required* to be MDs). Many homeopaths started out as medical doctors, nurse practitioners, pharmacists, chiropractors, or acupuncturists who wanted to add the power of homeopathy to the modalities they offer their clients. Others go directly to professional homeopathy training without going through conventional medical training first.

Either way, ideally they'll have the CCH credential (Certified Classical Homeopath, indicating the person is nationally certified after 1000 hours of training). Check **www.HomeopathicDirectory.org**. However, there are good homeopaths who do not have this credential, sometimes because they were already in practice when the credential was created 20 years ago, sometimes because their practice is so busy they don't feel the need for the credential. This is especially true of MD homeopaths. They are rare and you are lucky if you can find one.

There are only about 500 of us CCH-certified homeopaths in the United States, so you may need to use my fallback option for finding a homeopath: word of mouth.

### Working with Your Homeopath

Your homeopath will give you a "constitutional remedy," a single medicine individualized for you and meant to address your chronic illness plus improve your health overall. Some homeopaths feel that using "acute remedies" like those recommended in this book will interfere with your constitutional remedy. They may even recommend repeating your constitutional remedy any time you get sick, instead of the specific homeopathic medicines in this book. Some homeopaths will be fine with my vitamin-and-herb recommendations, while others will ask you not to take anything except their remedy.

Your homeopath may also ask you to abstain from things that might antidote the remedy, like coffee, mint, dental work, and electric blankets. There is a long tradition in homeopathy that these things may interfere, but many of us find that they don't. However, you should respect the requests of your professional homeopath. The results are likely to be worth it.

# THE JOURNEY CONTINUES

This has been quite a journey, hasn't it? I hope you've learned a lot about natural healing—and I hope you've tried some things for yourself. I know it's a lot all at once. How about this: make a promise to yourself that every time you dip into this book for a quick answer to a health crisis, you'll also flip through the first section to follow just one suggestion for a permanent change in your lifestyle.

Or maybe you'll be like Dagmar, a cheery grandmother who came into my health food store for advice on how to lose weight. It was a quiet Sunday afternoon and we talked for an hour, wandering far afield from her original question. She was open to all my suggestions, as she remembered the healthy lifestyle of her childhood on a farm in Germany.

Dagmar came back a month later, her cheeks rosy as apples. She had, that same day, stopped smoking, become a vegetarian, thrown out all the processed food from her pantry, begun a vigorous daily walking and weight loss routine, and started taking all the supplements I recommended. This retired museum curator embarked on a second career coaching others in switching to a healthy lifestyle.

For most people, these changes take time. Try one thing at a time. See what works. Seek out others to explore with. If there's no one in your immediate circle, look a little further afield. The interest in natural healing is sweeping the country and you are already a part of it.

## Expanding the Vision

If we can make these changes on a larger scale, we can have a healthier health care system. Right now our health care system is a sick patient indeed, "bleeding red ink" as our high-tech, highly invasive, after-it's-too-late approach siphons off precious resources. Health care costs are bankrupting individual families, exacerbating labor disputes, and sabotaging attempts to balance government budgets.

Why not start with the simplest, safest, and least-invasive method first whenever it's appropriate, before trying something more drastic? We could save so much money in our health care system this way. I love the vision for our health care system set forth in Dr. Len Saputo's book *A Return to Healing*. I recommend it to everyone and especially to my fellow health care practitioners, to health insurance executives, and to anyone involved with public policy regarding health care.

Dr. Saputo proposes treating people who have chronic illnesses first with good nutrition and exercise, then with no-harm, non-invasive natural therapies. If those methods don't work, he suggests using functional medicine (high-potency supplements) and only as a last resort, if all else fails, turning to drugs (used sparingly) and surgery. This approach makes me think of my father, the vascular surgeon, who would try to get his patients to stop smoking, start exercising, lose weight, and change their eating habits before he would operate on them.

Acute care (for recent, self-limiting, everyday complaints) can be triaged in the same way as well, and that's what this book is about. My vision is to help change health care in America by making this book easily available through employee wellness programs, health insurance companies, and practitioners' offices. If you're involved with any of these organizations, I invite you to get in touch with me.

## Keep In Touch

Readers are welcome to email me questions of general interest at **burke@YourNaturalMedicineCabinet.com** and I'll answer them in my blog on the same site. Let me know if you have favorite books, websites, or natural remedies that I haven't covered in this book. Let's take this journey of natural healing together!

# ACKNOWLEDGMENTS

This book began with the customers in my health food store and continued with my colleagues and clients at the Lydian Center for Innovative Medicine in Cambridge, Mass. I am grateful for my professional training to the Social Studies department at Harvard University, the nursing school at Quincy College, and my homeopathic mentors Dr. Luc De Schepper and Dr. Joel Kreisberg.

For information on other modalities I am indebted to:

- **Supplements:** Elizabeth Stagl of Cambridge Naturals in Cambridge, Mass. (**www.CambridgeNaturals.com**). Elizabeth and her husband Michael Kanter generously shared their knowledge with me when I opened my store in 1977.
- **Chiropractic:** Lydia Knutson, DC of the Lydian Center for Innovative Medicine, **www.LydianCenter.com.**
- **Craniosacral:** Eve Kodiak, MM of the Lydian Center for Innovative Medicine, **www.EveKodiak.com.**
- **Flower essences:** Donna Thompson, certified spiritual counselor and energy intuitive, **findsacredjoy@aol.com.**

As for creating this book, I owe endless thanks to my agent and expert publishing consultant, Nigel J. Yorwerth, who envisioned the book long before I could have imagined it and prodded me to create it. Nigel Yorwerth and Patricia Spadaro of Yorwerth Associates/ PublishingCoaches.com gave me invaluable feedback and guidance and have been the midwives to this book at every step through its long but gratifying birthing process, assisting me with everything from editing and design to marketing, distribution, and foreign rights sales.

I owe the greatest debt of gratitude to my sainted parents, who gave me the funds they had set aside for my medical school tuition so that I could open a health food store instead.

# NOTES, REFERENCES
# AND THE FINE PRINT

A complete set of references could be twice as long as the book itself. I have limited these notes to supportive information and precautions. Additional notes, bibliographical references, and links to all the websites referenced may be found at www.YourNaturalMedicineCabinet.com

**page 11, Dr. Terry Wahls' TED Talk:** Search for Terry Wahls on YouTube and you'll find this astounding video, which shows her before (in a wheelchair) and after (walking around just fine as she delivers the talk). Dr. Wahls, as a department head in a university hospital, was given the "nothing more we can do for you" verdict by conventional medicine, then did her own research on how to reverse MS naturally.

**page 12, the dangers of microwaves:** from *The Proven Dangers of Microwaves* on Dr. Mercola's site, www.Mercola.com/article/microwave/hazards2.htm, which in turn is extracted from *NEXUS Magazine*, Volume 2, #25 (April-May 1995). The sources listed in this article include:

- The Minnesota Extension Service of the University of Minnesota (recommending not to microwave baby bottles because of the loss of some vitamins and protective properties).
- A lawsuit from the family of a woman who died after surgery because she received blood warmed in a microwave, demonstrating how microwaving can alter the properties of a substance.
- A study in the November 2003 issue of *The Journal of the Science of Food and Agriculture* showing that microwaved broccoli lost up to 97% of its antioxidants compared to 11% lost when steamed.
- A study done by a Swiss food scientist who demonstrated alarming changes in the health of previously robust people (from the Macrobiotic Institute) after only a few days on microwaved foods.

Worth a read. If this is what they knew about 15 years ago, think of how much more is known now.

**page 13, my busy colleague who advised parents not to microwave their baby formula:** This was my highly respected colleague Dr. Tinus Smits, the Dutch doctor who wrote *Autism Beyond Despair*. He had many recommendations for a healthier lifestyle, including avoiding the use of a microwave. *Autism Beyond Despair* is worth buying just for its healthy lifestyle recommendations — then consider giving it to a family with an autistic child. Dr. Smits developed a method for reversing the symptoms of autism, and he had 300 cured cases (or well on the way to cure) when he passed away in 2010. Dr. Smits trained homeopaths in the Netherlands and the US who are using his method successfully. See www. Cease-Therapy.com.

**page 23, multivitamins:** Men and non-menstruating women should avoid vitamins containing **iron. Copper** is necessary but only in small amounts (1 mg or less). Avoid multivitamins with 2 mg or more of copper.

**page 24, Vitamin D:** Home vitamin D tests are available from **www. VitaminDCouncil.org.** Get your blood level tested in the winter when it's likely to be low, not in the summer when sun exposure brings it to a peak. If you are really deficient in D, you can raise your blood level quickly by taking 10,000 IU a day, but only do this short term. Either plan to test your blood level again or plan on dropping back to 5,000 IU a day after three months. Doctors typically refer to the recent guidelines from the Institute of Medicine (IOM) which recommend much lower levels of vitamin D, but most vitamin D experts disagree with the IOM guidelines.

Definitely don't get the vitamin D shot with 50,000 IU because it contains D2, not D3. D2 is not only relatively ineffective, it can even be harmful. If you're buying your vitamin D in a health food store, you don't need to read the label, because health food store brands all use D3.

The vitamin D created on your skin when exposed to sunlight is really the best form of all. Ideally get an hour a day of sunlight without sunscreen on your skin. If you would like to imitate the effect of sunlight but are stuck in the office all day, get the best sun lamp, the one used in research on vitamin D: the Sperti KBD-UV lamp, available online from **www.Sperti.com.**

Vitamin D is safe for pregnant and lactating women, according to research conducted by Dr. Bruce Hollis, the acknowledged expert on Vitamin D.

**page 24, calcium and magnesium recommendations:** While the official recommendation is for 1200 mg of calcium, that figure includes what we get from food, and most people in the US get enough calcium from food that we can reduce our need for supplementation. People who avoid dairy products can still get plenty of calcium from green leafy vegetables, beans (including tofu and other soy products), and sesame tahini, which makes just about any food more wonderful. Think about it: if calcium is in milk, the cows must have gotten it from somewhere—from eating their green vegetables!

The absolute amount of calcium in the diet is less important than the many factors that cause the body to store or excrete calcium, as explained briefly in the Osteoporosis section and at great length in Pam Levin's *Perfect Bones*. You need to adjust the amount of calcium you take, depending on these factors.

The Pioneer formula features microcrystalline calcium hydroxyapatite, a superexcellent source of calcium plus other substances needed for strong bones.

As for magnesium, you might notice in this book's Index of Recommendations that magnesium is recommended for many different health conditions, because it's one of the most crucial deficiencies in our diet, unless you're really a champ at eating those green vegetables or downing your green smoothies. And actually those greens have to be organic, from well-composted soil, because our conventional produce comes from mineral-deficient soil.

While the conventional wisdom is that we need twice as much calcium as magnesium, we need to supplement magnesium more carefully because the SAD (Standard American Diet) is so magnesium-deficient.

**page 26, Vitamin D recommendations for children:** Kids need to get out in the sun without sunscreen! Half an hour a day is a good amount. Kids spend too much time inside with their electronics; see the "Get Strength from Nature" chapter. Then if they do go out, parents are so afraid of skin cancer that they keep kids constantly slathered with sunscreens (which contain carcinogenic chemicals, unless you check the ingredients carefully at Environmental Working Group's Sunscreen Guide, **www.EWG.org**). The lack of sun exposure is causing an epidemic of rickets (soft bones from a vitamin D deficiency), a disease that supposedly disappeared along with the tenements of the 19th century. But these are well-fed middle class kids, which has everyone alarmed. As to how to give kids Vitamin D, good brands include Carlson's Vitamin D drops for babies and for children, and Nature's Plus berry-flavored chewable vitamin D for kids.

**page 47, febrile seizures considered benign:** For example, the Mayo Clinic website acknowledges how "alarming" febrile seizures can be for parents (the kids go unconscious and tremble or shake all over), but reassures them that "the vast majority of febrile seizures cause no lasting effects." It recommends protecting small children having a seizure by loosening tight clothing and holding them or laying them down to prevent injury (**www.MayoClinic.com**, do a search for febrile seizures).

**page 76, fermented foods like kefir and miso:** Fermented foods have been traditional foods around the world since time immemorial because they keep well without refrigeration and have many added health benefits. They are easier to digest than their unfermented versions because the fermenting microbes have partly broken them down, and the microbes also create vitamins and enzymes that our bodies need. Kefir is a fermented milk drink like a liquid yogurt but made from a different starter culture (kefir grains), while miso is a fermented soy paste traditionally used as a soup base in Japan. Sauerkraut is a more familiar food in the US, but it has to be fresh, not bottled, for its precious enzymes to be intact.

**page 89, double tall skinny vanilla:** If you're like me and never go into Starbucks, you probably need a translation. In Starbucks-speak, this means a small coffee (Starbucks calls it a "tall" so they can charge more) with skim milk, vanilla flavoring and an extra shot of espresso.

**page 96, Urtica urens tincture for gout:** This was the secret formula of Dr. James Compton Burnett, a 19th century homeopath who became famous as "Dr. Gout" because of his success in treating this disease of upper class Brits who ate too much beef. His prescription was five drops of the tincture in a wineglassful of warm water every two or three hours. The herbal formula made the urine more plentiful, dark, and loaded with uric acid, relieving the inflamed joints.

**page 128, Gaia Herb's Liver Support:** This formula is meant to be taken every day, while their more intense **Liver Cleanse** is used intermittently, typically twice a year for two weeks at a time.

**page 128, Terry Naturally Curamed Curcumin:** This is a very special formula that makes the curcumin easily absorbed and used by your body. Curcumin (the active ingredient in turmeric) is pretty much inert by itself, but this special extract developed in India brings out curcumin's ability to detoxify the liver, reduce inflammation, and even reduce the plaques associated with Alzheimer's. Terry Naturally is the only brand with this special patented form of curcumin.

**page 145, "vision walk":** This concept came from my colleague, the late Dr. Antonia Orfield, a behavioral optometrist who used eye exercises, nutrition and homeopathy in her practice at Harvard University Health Services. It was her observation that developing peripheral vision also helps the brain to hold the "big picture" instead of becoming overfocused on details. In fact, she had a client who was nearsighted and whom she helped to develop peripheral vision. He credited her with his being able to finish his doctoral dissertation because he was now able to "see" the overall scope of his idea instead of just "looking at" the details.

**page 155, the energetic template or blueprint of the body:** For more about this concept, see *Vibrational Medicine* by Richard Gerber and *Energy Medicine: The Scientific Basis* by James Oschman and Candace Pert.

**page 172, water retention or excessive dryness:** Did you know that puffiness, for example in your ankles or in your fingers so your rings don't fit, can be a sign of dehydration? People tend to think of water retention as a sign that they have drunk too much water so they stop, but actually the opposite is the case. The body is very smart, and when you get dehydrated it starts to hold on to its water.

If you're dehydrated, it's best not to gulp a lot of water quickly nor to use sports drinks (electrolyte-replacement drinks). When your stomach fills up with water quickly, it sends a message to the kidneys, "Lots of fluid coming in! Crank up the output!" and that's why it seems that the more you drink, the quicker you pee it all out. Frustrating, isn't it? Sip slowly for better retention.

You do need salt and trace minerals to go with all that water. Sports drinks are a poor source, though—health-wise because of their artificial ingredients and economically because of the cost of shipping all that water and glass. Instead, replace trace minerals directly. You can get electrolyte mineral replacements at your health food store or get all the minerals you need from sea vegetables. One of the favorite supplements among my fellow marathoners is dulse, a sea vegetable. Spread the little clumps into thin leaves for easy chewing or (my favorite) sauté in melted butter to make dulse chips. Use Nat. mur. cell salt at the same time.

**page 183, top fashion models:** Chang, Bee-Shyuan. "Skin Deep: Seeking Relief through Arnica," *New York Times,* Sept. 15, 2011.

**page 216, homeopathy works on animals:** Homeopathy shows promise in enabling farmers to reduce the use of antibiotics in animals, thereby minimizing public health concerns with antibiotics in the waterways and antibiotic-resistant bacteria. As a bonus, homeopathic treatment is much less expensive for the farmer. For example, recent research in Germany demonstrated that a homeopathic remedy combination was as effective as antibiotics in preventing the piglet version of kennel cough. Other studies have shown that mastitis in dairy cows can be treated by putting remedies in their watering trough (so much for the belief that remedies require distilled water!) and that remedies can reduce stillbirth in pigs and complications of birth among dairy cows. References in *Homeopathic Family Medicine,* an eBook by Dana Ullman (www.Homeopathic.com).

**page 216, homeopathy works on plants:** A whole new field of homeopathy has recently sprouted, so to speak, in Europe and Australia based on using homeopathy for plants. Homeopathic medicines can be used to treat diseased plants, to fend off pests, to improve blossoming of flowering plants and the flavor of fruits, and to enhance the absorption of nutrients in weak, sickly plants. The original work in the field, *Homeopathy for Farm and Garden* by Vaikunthanath das Kaviraj, is thorough and authoritative but a bit difficult to understand for anyone not already versed in homeopathy. The newer *Homeopathy for Plants* by Christiane Maute is full of helpful information easily accessible for the amateur gardener and homeopathic newbie alike. (Both available from www.Minimum.com.)

**page 218, regulated as drugs by the FDA:** All the common homeopathic medicines available in stores are considered over-the-counter drugs by the FDA. Just as conventional medicines approved by the FDA are listed in the USP (United States Pharmacopeia), so too homeopathic medicines approved by the FDA are listed in the HPUS (the Homeopathic Pharmacopeia of the US). The FDA inspects the facilities that manufacture homeopathic medicines and insists on certain standards for their production. This close oversight of homeopathic medicines is entirely different from the FDA's arms-length approach to vitamins, minerals, herbs and other supplements, based on a lesser degree of regulatory authority granted by Congress.

**page 229, testing yourself by using applied kinesiology:** Kinesiology, also known as muscle testing, muscle monitoring, and muscle biofeedback, provides access to the subconscious because muscles directly access the subconscious parts of the brain. When the muscle being tested "locks" or feels strong, this indicates that there are no active stressors affecting the person being tested. When the person is stressed, the muscle's contraction is inhibited and it "unlocks" (feels weak). Muscle biofeedback can access different kinds of stress at different levels within the person, including emotional, structural and biochemical. For a review of the scientific research documenting the accuracy and effectiveness of muscle biofeedback, consult the textbook *Fundamentals of Energetic Kinesiology* (Krebs & McGowan, forthcoming, 2013).

**page 241, interest in natural healing is sweeping the country:** Actually the trend was noted 20 years ago in a landmark study by Dr. David Eisenberg at Harvard Medical School. It shocked the medical community by revealing that Americans were making more visits to providers of "unconventional therapies" than to their primary care doctors, spending more than ten billion dollars out of pocket in the process, and for the most part not telling their doctors about it. Eisenberg DM, Kessler RC, Foster C, Norlock F, Calkins DR, Delbanco TL. Unconventional medicine in the United States—prevalence, costs, and patterns of use. *N Engl J Med* 1993; 328:246-252.

# INDEX OF CONDITIONS

# INDEX OF RECOMMENDATIONS

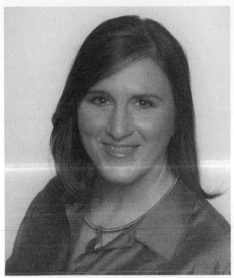

Photo by Savas Studios

Burke Lennihan RN, CCH has spent over 30 years in different aspects of holistic health care. She currently practices classical homeopathy at the Lydian Center for Innovative Medicine in Cambridge, Mass.

After graduating from Harvard University at the top of her class, she opened and operated health food stores in Boston and Cambridge for 16 years, where she developed her expertise in natural remedies. In 1996, she cofounded and administered the Renaissance Institute of Classical Homeopathy with her mentor, internationally distinguished homeopath Dr. Luc De Schepper. She subsequently directed Teleosis School of Homeopathy from 2002 to 2009.

Lennihan is a health expert on Dr. Mehmet Oz's ShareCare.com and is also the producer and host of the local TV show *A Healer In Every Home*, available on the GreenHealingTV channel on YouTube. She has also written and coauthored several books and articles on natural health. With more than 35 years of experience in meditation, she teaches classes in heart-center meditation at Harvard University's Center for Wellness and is a lecturer on holistic health at Massachusetts College of Pharmacy and Lesley University. To learn more about Burke Lennihan and her work, visit **www.YourNaturalMedicineCabinet.com**.